THE

CARNIVORE

DIET

AN ANCESTRAL RESET TO OPTIMAL HUMAN HEALTH

By Kurt Yazici

To my incredible team at Crushvertise @crushvertise,who have stuck by me as their leader and supported this often, "wild" mission. Matt, Eli, John, Ralph, Louis, I appreciate you all so much for all that you do and your continued dedication to excellence.

To my grandmother Jan Karner, who battled schizophrenia for 4 decades before passing away Jan 1st, 2018. Mental illness impacts so many of us, but there is real hope through diet and lifestyle changes. Especially as we continue to dissect and understand the root cause of disease, I'm grateful to be a part of this community and for the entire movement in functional health and wellness.

TABLE OF
CONTENTS

1. FOREWORD

Like so many of us, when I first heard about the carnivore diet, it sounded totally crazy to me. A diet without any plant foods- how could that possibly be healthy for humans? How would I poop without fiber? What about polyphenols and their supposed anti-oxidant properties? Would I get sick of eating meat every day?

For so much of my life, I too had been admonished to "eat my fruit and vegetables." It was incredibly challenging at first to look past this conditioning and my cognitive biases to examine the carnivore diet with an open mind.

But many of you reading this already know where this story leads. I did explore the carnivore diet, and I did it intensely. Over the last two years, researching the nuances of this way of eating has occupied almost all of my waking hours. Even when I've been in the ocean chasing that perfect wave, thoughts about plant toxins, micronutrients, and the incredible potential of regenerative agriculture to heal the earth have been marinating in my meat-fueled brain.

During the past two years, I've also lived the carnivore diet, and what I have experienced first hand has been nothing short of amazing. Profound improvements in mood, energy and mental clarity were surprising positive effects of this way of eating, but a complete resolution of severe eczema has been the most striking benefit of this way of eating.

Amazingly, stories like mine are not unique. As word about the benefits of an animal-based diet continues to spread like wildfire, more and more people are finding similar benefits from this way of eating. It now appears undeniable that lives are being changed for the better every single day by the carnivore diet.

As you'll read in this book, Kurt's story is yet another illustration of this, and I'm so glad he's decided to share it with the world in these pages. We've known each other for a number of years, first crossing paths about 3 years ago amidst mutual interests in health and optimal performance at a gym in Seattle when he had a lot less beard and a lot longer hair. He's gone from "Fabio Kurt" to "Lumberjack Kurt" in my eyes. Kurt is a dashing guy with both looks, but this physical transition has been accompanied by significant health improvements coupled with his own carnivore journey. Longstanding stomach issues have disappeared with the elimination of plants, as did his previously challenging anxiety, depression and skin issues.

How can this be? How can the elimination of plants, and the emphasis on animal meat and organs result in such marked improvements in health for Kurt, me, and thousands of others who have discovered the carnivore diet? Though many of these ideas fly in the face of conventional wisdom, you'll soon discover that we've been badly misled with regard to nutritional dogma.

As Kurt will discuss in this book, though plants are beautiful to look at, they aren't as benign as we've been led to believe, and they certainly don't want to be eaten. Throughout their co-evolution with animals for the last 450 million years plants have developed myriad toxins to defend themselves, and these can be quite damaging for many individuals. We've also been misled about meat. Animal foods are, in fact, incredibly nutritious, and an indispensable part of the human diet. Studies painting meat in a negative light are invariably of the observational epidemiology sort, and cannot be used to make causative inferences. They can only be used to make hypotheses which must then be put to the test with interventional studies. When the latter types of studies are done we discover something striking: meat of all kinds is good for humans, not bad for us!

I'm so excited for you to learn more about the carnivore diet by reading this book. Being able to think critically and remain open minded allows us all to grow. Challenging old ideas is sometimes difficult for us but it is the only way forward if we hope to avoid stagnation.

Stay Radical!
Paul Saladino, MD
Author of The Carnivore Code
carnivoremd.com

2. PREFACE

Welcome, I'm deeply excited for you and your commitment to learning this way of eating and living. *I went from literally suffering, to absolutely thriving. From a place of rock bottom - physically and emotionally stuck, to a place now where I am facing and overcoming my greatest challenges with true resilience and vitality.*

The incredible part is that for many of you, this isn't about improving what you're currently doing. But instead, about changing your trajectory and heading off in a completely different direction.

This book is a summary of everything I've learned along my Carnivore Diet journey. There may be sections you wish to skip, and that's absolutely fine. Use it as a reference, as a tool to get where you want to go. In writing this I was challenged to answer many of the most common thoughts and concerns I once had. Some of these will be more interesting and relevant, while others may not.

I've laid out the book by starting with my personal story. I then explain the Carnivore Diet, how and why it works. I go on to discuss why one would want to do it, and then exactly how to do it. I finish with several cases and conditions from which we've seen tremendous anecdotal evidence of treatment through this way of eating.

You can read from start to finish or you can simply jump to sections you find most relevant to your interests. Use the table of contents to direct you to the sections you prefer.

I want to thank you for investing in learning about your health. In spite of its fame of a statement, ignorance is not bliss. Though, it can be painful - I believe diving into what hurts one self and tackling the source is the most rewarding thing one can do.

3. MY JOURNEY
INTO CARNIVORE

I wouldn't be here if it weren't for a tremendous story that deeply impacted my life. This is the story of how I discovered the Carnivore Diet and how all of this came to be. all of this came to be.

2014

I was nervous and relieved all at once. I'd just quit my near decade long corporate career and I'd plummeted full-on into entrepreneurship. I'd been attempting to launch a "side hustle" ever since I read The 4-Hour Workweek by Tim Ferris. But the demands and pull of my corporate careers kept my energy focused largely on their demands.

After a few half-hearted attempts, I finally decided the only way I was going to make it was to "burn the boats" and make success my only option. I'd saved up enough of a nest egg to generate around 12 months of "runway" to start my venture. I knew

if all else failed I could lean back on my resume and family to find a way back to earning an income.

While this was happening I'd been following Tim Ferris, the author of The 4-Hour Workweek and Dave Asprey, CEO and founder of Bulletproof. The prior year I'd grown a strong passion for self-optimization and felt these authors were leading the way. I'd started experimenting with Bulletproof and ketogenic diets. My breakfasts were quite enjoyable. As a newly minted "entrepreneur" I'd wake up and french press a delicious "bulletproof coffee" which was composed of grass fed butter and mct oil. But before we go further, let's back up for a moment.

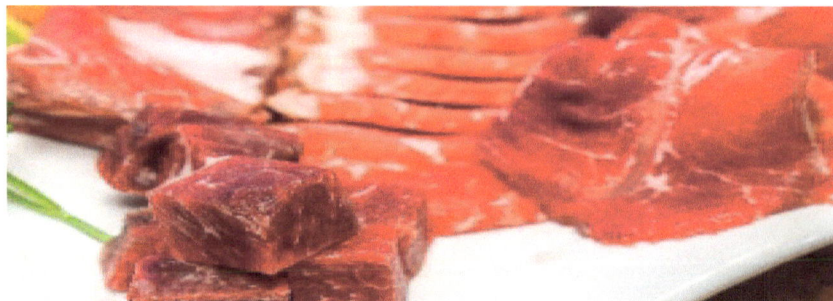

Image: freepik.com

1995, (11 y/o) Childhood Gut issues

As a kid growing up I had major acne, gut and anxiety issues. I would have loose stools, bloating and gut cramping weekly. Thinking back it always followed a meal or drink. Dinner at Grandma's house might have me struggling to make it back in the car ride home.

My gut never felt at ease, and it transferred into the way I felt socially. I'd usually do okay with breakfast - often eating cereal with skim milk or eggs and toast. Lunch at school was often cracker pizza or cheese burgers and fries along with apple juice or a side of chocolate milk. Surprisingly, I did well at school in terms of gut issues, but by the end of dinner I would often find myself not feeling well.

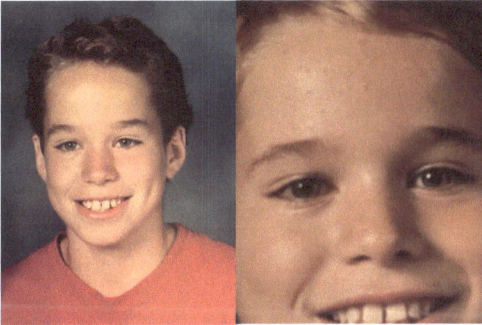

Image: Kurt's Youth and Acne approaching early teens

1997, (13 y/o) Skin, Acne

Once I hit my teens my skin got real. Nasty! I developed some of the most embarrassing oily acne skin you'd see. I didn't worry too much about it - it was normal for a lot of kids to have it. But as I headed further into my teens my acne got to a point where I started seeing a dermatologist. After trying a slew of different over-the-counter regimens I started taking prescription retinol and Differin gels.

These didn't help much and ultimately I was placed on Accutane. This dried me out from the inside. I would get nose bleeds and dry throat and feel the lack of mucus in my body. But it definitely helped my acne and after 6 months taking it my skin really cleared up! I wouldn't recommend this for anyone though, there are some serious side effects and to this day *I'm fairly certain it permanently damaged my sense of smell.* Some people experience hearing, vision and other irreversible internal organ damage.

I believe my Accutane use contributed significantly to 70-80% loss of my sense of smell along with a 20 years later sinus surgery to clear out blockage in my sinuses from scarring that occurred from the dryness. That said, at the time it did treat my skin situation quite effectively. The embarrassment started to lift and I felt more "normal." Side note - Little did I know simply cutting out dairy could do wonders for my skin.

Back to my youth. Those pesky gut issues continued. My loving parents tried to help me. I went and saw several doctors and specialists. Blood tests along with some very uncomfortable physical exams yielded no pathogens or clear causes at the time.

As I grew into my teens I became less picky on eating for flavor and got a better sense of what I could eat and not eat to avoid issues. There wasn't much of an internet, let alone gut health information available. We all just "knew" fat, red meat and cholesterol were bad. Many people who ate those foods were much sicker than people who didn't.

2006 Anxiety

I made it through high school living fairly well within my comfort zone. I went on to college to study pre-med. In my sophomore year I had my first anxiety attack. I was sitting in my professor's office talking to him and I just started sweating profusely. *This totally freaked me out. It was the first time I'd created physical symptoms of anxiety with my thoughts.* I really hadn't thought much about my diet or gut, but now I was keenly aware of how I felt in terms of if I was anxious, or potentially thinking about anxiety.

If you've ever had significant anxiety you'll know that it becomes a vicious cycle of fearing the symptoms and often more intensely the fear itself. A condition that only gets more intense if not checked and properly treated.

Those anxious sensations can be truly crippling and terrifying. I vividly remember the moment, all of a sudden heating up and sweating, as my heart started beating out of my chest. As I focused on those sensations taking me over, I didn't realize I was actually amplifying them over and over by thinking about them.

Anxiety is the most common mental illness, affecting 40M Americans. [51] I believe many people struggle with varying degrees of anxiety and never truly conquer it their entire lives. It can be tough to diagnose and treat, as it often manifests deeply in avoidance habits. You completely avoid the events that may potentially trigger the start of it, as such symptoms only come on if you're "caught" in a situation you're not ready for.

The Cycle of Anxiety

Anxiety

Long term: Building sensations of anxious symptoms

Short term: Increased intensity of symptoms and avoidance of triggers

Relief

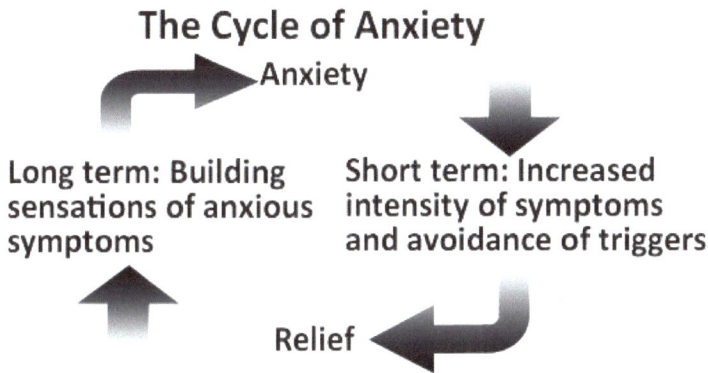

Since I would sweat and get overheated, that meant I always had to wear light, breathable clothing, and avoid rooms and situations where I thought I might get too hot. It also meant avoiding situations where stress could get too high and I'd feel like I couldn't "escape." Public speaking, presenting, even grocery lines all qualified as situations I did much to avoid. Years later I would learn more about the psychological aspects - read several texts - seek out counseling and make great steps towards facing the things I was avoiding.

I intend to write a text on anxiety. Join my newsletter to learn more about when this will be coming out.

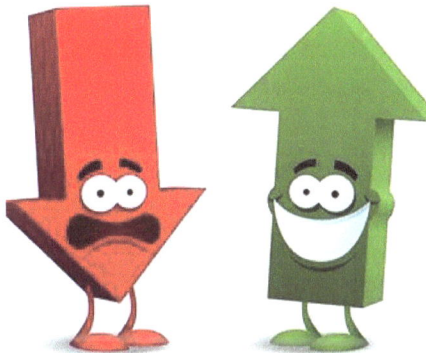

2014-2015

While I was learning how I was going to build my "business," and create an online income, I'd become fascinated in improving my mental and physical performance. I'd been living in NYC and decided to move back in with my family to save money while I was bootstrapping my company. Bulletproof coffee, a keto diet and low-carb products became a lifestyle for me. I was learning affiliate marketing and focusing on Facebook ads. My hobby became exploring and learning about my diet optimization.

I'd been a couple years into drinking bulletproof coffee and intermittent fasting (IF). I'd break the fast mid-morning with Bulletproof and Quest bars, with a later keto diet of some variation of meat, eggs, cheese and avocado. In my afternoons I'd whip up one of these "super-smoothies" with almond butter and continue into the evening with my day.

I'd met Dr. Paul Saladino (CarnivoreMD) at the local rock climbing gym in Seattle where we'd both spend daily afternoons getting movement and sauna time. At this time neither of us knew anything about the Carnivore diet, but I knew Paul was becoming a Psychiatrist and getting certified to be a Functional MD.

We were both active and passionate about wellness and optimization. He became a great friend and my go-to doc. I'd also started following more podcasts and "thought-leaders" like Rhonda Patrick. Her information introduced me to the idea of consuming "powerful" antioxidants and xenohermetics. Consuming "superfoods" like kale, spinach, broccoli sprouts, chia seeds and almond butter to get such nutrients.

2016

My young business had been surviving, but had yet to thrive. We'd consistently post months with losses after profits. It was emotionally draining to experience the joy of earning $50K one month only to lose it all the following month.

Looking back I realized we'd overgrown who I was as a leader. A year prior I'd (I was 31 at the time) had brought on a younger (19) brother to be a part owner. I'd built a team of six employees in Seattle and another dozen overseas. In addition, neither of us were truly passionate about the product and process of the business, we found ourselves working simply to earn money.

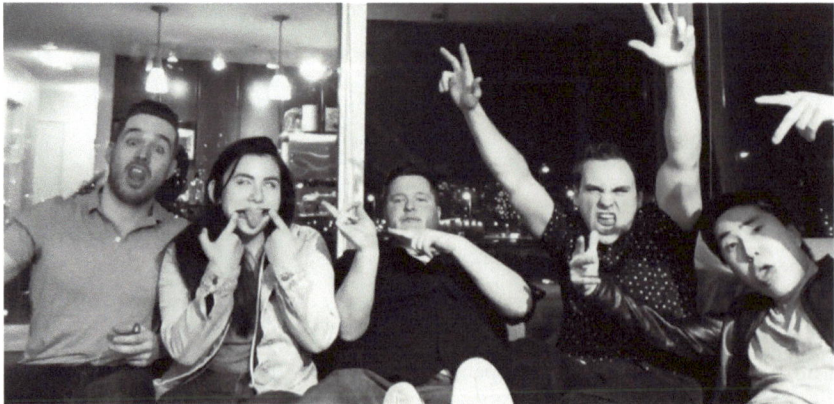

Image: Early Crushvertise Team in March 2016

As we went through challenges, we began to struggle more to communicate, and became increasingly frustrated and irritated with each other. As this was happening, a low level of anxiety started growing within me. That feeling got me thinking that the keto diet and lifestyle were negatively affecting my cardiovascular health and causing this tension and stress I was experiencing in my chest.

While this was happening, I'd started dating a lady that was emotionally and physically unhealthy for me. Late nights, alcohol and often unpredictable scheduling all lead to more anxiety and added stress.

All this piled onto our wobbly business profits and very low cash reserves, growing tensions between my brother and me, ultimately reaching a breaking point.

2016 Panic Attack

One day it all came crashing down. Sitting in the office at my desk I had a terrifying panic attack. I was sitting there angry, scared, frustrated and literally thought I was having a stroke or a heart attack.

I started feeling light-headed, my heart was pounding, my chest tightening, I was getting dizzy. I went upstairs to lie down and messaged my team to let them know I wasn't feeling well. That experience scared the crap out of me. After a couple hours, and feeling a bit more manageable, I walked a few blocks up the street to the urgent care.

They ran a few tests, checked my heart rate and blood pressure and asked me a series of cardiovascular diagnostic questions. The nurse practitioner came back after getting the test results. I'll never forget what she said to me, "You just have anxiety." She then proceeded to prescribe me prescription beta-blockers to mask the symptoms.

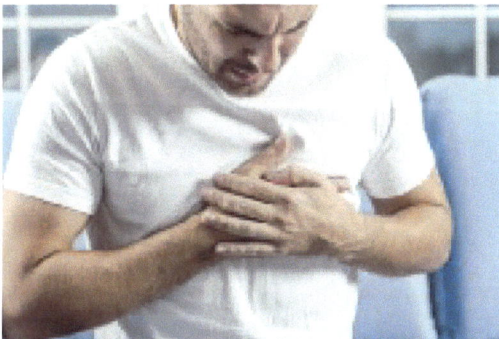

image: freepik.com

Numbing Medication

This experience totally rocked me and my nervous system. Anxiety had become so intense at this point that I didn't want to take or do anything that would limit my "control" or feelings of ease. I found myself going up to the break room we had every couple of hours to try out different Neuro Linguistic Programming (NLP) and mind techniques to counter the anxious feelings that would build up while sitting in my office.

I felt the anxiety build whenever I sat in the office. It became a challenge to go for a walk outside. I'd start walking, feel my heart rate increase and experience so much fear thinking I was going to experience another debilitating anxious moment.

I felt so anxious, but really didn't want to take drugs to block the anxiety. I was determined not to numb myself, but instead figure out what was at the source of all the anxiety. I really just wanted to feel better. Emotionally though **I felt very stuck**. I think this is the hardest place for someone to be.

When you experience emotional pain but it's not constant, you at least have a sense of hope that it will change. But when you are in a state of a constant perpetual anxious climb with limited relief, there's very little to look forward to. Business was struggling, my relationships with my team were struggling and I eventually ended the relationship I was in. Anxiety was constant.

Through all of this I did manage to stay away from toxic habits of drugs and alcohol and I did keep going to the gym. I found relief with sauna, cold winter showers and exercise. Those activities would shift my physiology and minimize the anxiety for a

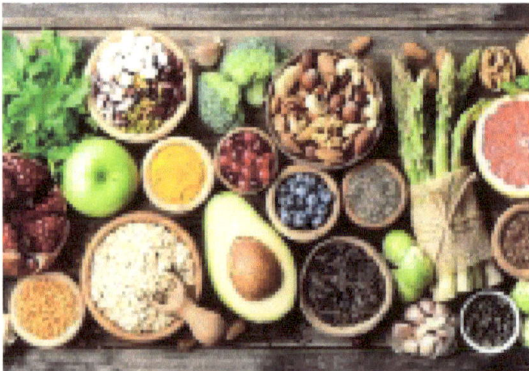

Image: https://www.rd.com/food/superfoods-nutritionists-eat-in-fall/

brief period. I also noticed moments while watching films or playing soccer, where I'd get completely out of the anxiety pattern before slipping back in.

While this was going on my diet and bulletproof consumption were still my priority. To be frank, they were my main joy and pleasure at the time. Deep down I was thinking that getting my "superfoods" and super smoothies of kale, broccoli sprouts, spinach, almond butter, local honey, cacao nibs, flax seeds, blueberries and cinnamon was saving my health and me. It was delicious and I was convinced I was optimizing myself by consuming them.

2017 Winter

Then one day I woke up and I felt physically cold and down. I'd never experienced this feeling before. I was cold physically, and felt a deep sense of fear and sadness. I later learned this is one way in which depression can manifest and I had never experienced it first hand. My battle with anxiety and lack of positive progress had dragged me into a state of depression.

Looking for answers, I'd started reading a lot about anxiety. I read everything I could find on the topic. A friend had turned me on to a book "The Happiness Trap" by Russ Harris. The book really resonated with me and taught the A.C.T. Therapy philosophy.

I decided to seek a professional who knew this line of therapy. After several months of weekly sessions and some painful discussions, we made some real progress. I learned more about my mental patterns and how they were tripping me up and holding me back.

The process was challenging. I'd often spend an hour before and after each session preparing my notes and thoughts. I really wanted to understand and come with thoughts and insights during our time together.

I'm very fortunate that during all this, I always prioritized exercise and diet and never had a desire to consume any substances that could numb me, even in the toughest of times. I'd known the benefits and value of staying active and eating a "healthy" diet. Everything I read told me that exercise was a great way to combat mental health. All the literature I was studying suggested veggies and diverse superfoods added tremendous health benefits.

Transition to Carnivore

Paul, my good friend and now @carnivoremd, and I connected largely through shared interest in learning about nutrition and diet. At the time he was doing consults and labs working with some of the folks at our gym - ordering blood panels and advising them on nutrition and supplementation.

After talking with him about some of my struggles we decided to do a consultation. We ran a full general review of bloodwork, added in a GI map and went through a slew of things to see if there was anything physical that stood out.

Secretly, I'd hoped something might be wrong so I could have an exact reason for all that had been happening to me physically and emotionally. But there wasn't anything out of the ordinary from my labs, and fortunately no gut pathogens came up either.

I shared some of the personal challenges and discussed the anxiety I was feeling. At the time neither of us knew about the Carnivore Diet, but Paul did have a feeling nutrition and diet might be a factor.

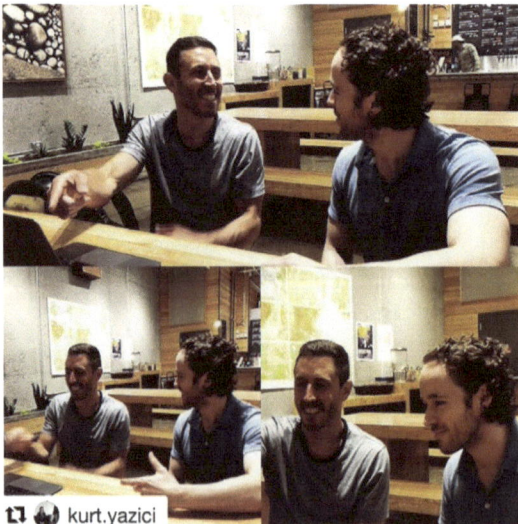

carnivoremd • Following

carnivoremd It's awesome to be able to work with superstar clients like this! Excited to continue this work. 🙌🔥 #Repost @kurt.yazici
. . .

Over the past couple of months I've started working with a functional medicine M.D. @paulsaladinomd Dr. Saladino has instrumental in helping me get a better sense of my genetics, and biomarkers to see where optimizations and corrections can be made.
If you're being prescribed meds to mask symptoms rather than explore and treat the sources AND your doctor isn't fitter than you, it may time for a change! "Today is the oldest you've ever been and the youngest you'll ever be again." Take

Liked by paulhwangmedia and 76 others
JUNE 12, 2018

Add a comment...

🔁 kurt.yazici

Image: Consult with my man Paul June 2018

Summer 2018

About this time CarnivoreMD had watched the Joe Rogan - Jordan Peterson interview on Youtube discussing how his daughter had gone into remission after decades of struggling with autoimmune and mental health issues. By her mid 20s she had multiple joint replacement surgeries due to her rheumatoid arthritis and struggle with debilitating depression.

After a couple of weeks seeing Paul in the gym he started promoting the Carnivore Diet more and more my way. One day Paul said, "I think you should try this Carnivore Diet thing." I was skeptical and apprehensive. He mentioned that his mood had shifted almost overnight, though he'd never dealt with major mental health issues, he immediately noticed a lift in how he felt.

I figured it was worth a shot to give this "Carnivore" thing a run. Paul and I were talking almost daily and he was experimenting with ways to eat. I slowly started transitioning into becoming full on Carnivore.

The rest is, as they say, history.

In the first 90 days (I slowly transitioned to full-on Carnivore after 1.5 - 2 months) I completely transformed my gut, skin, mood, energy, vitality and outlook on life. During that time my life stresses and work challenges did not diminish. In fact, we encountered many, all while moving my entire life and company across the country.

I'm truly excited you've taken this plunge. This is a totally new and (as Paul would say) radical way of eating and living and I'm honored to be your guide on this journey.

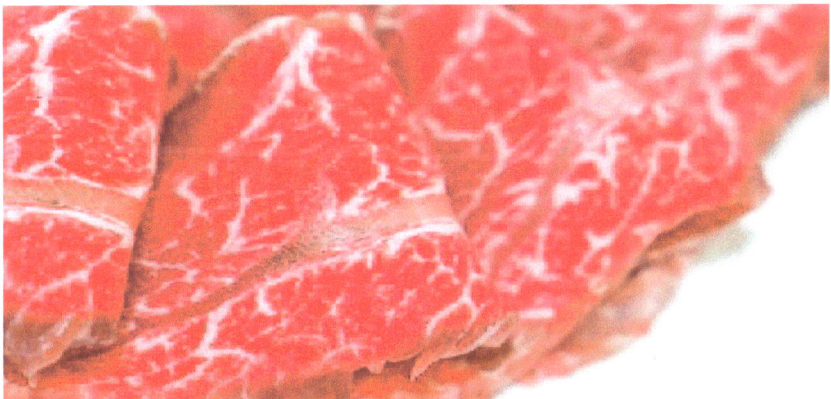

Image: freepik.com

Introduction of Carnivore Diet

It took me roughly 18 months of experimenting, trialing, tweaking and testing the diet to get to a level I felt consistent. During the beginning timeframe I went deeper into my biochemistry and biology. I've now done three rounds of blood work combined with urine, stool, and genetics testing. I introduced and removed foods, read, researched and self-educated through hours upon hours of studies and articles.

Week by week, through trial and error of personal testing, seeing what worked and how it impacted my markers, I became confident and at ease with this way of eating.

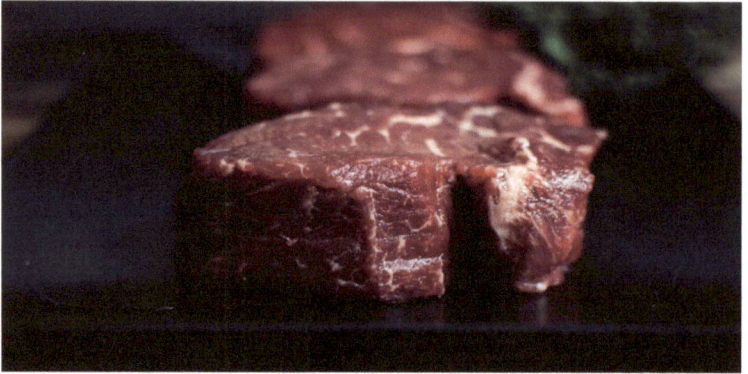

Image: freepik.com

Gut Ease

This diet completely transformed my gut issues. I went from always having a level of discomfort - leading to anxiety and dis-ease following meals, to completely forgetting what that feels like!

Anxiety

When I first started reading and working with professionals and counselors, diet was never discussed. Most advised against stimulants and drugs but the concept of foods being the trigger wasn't seen as primary lever to healing.

The reality is, anxiety can be greatly reduced by reducing certain foods. Most days I wake up feeling at ease. When I do get a spurt of energy it's less of the anxious nature and much more aligned with that of excitement. That default mood I start with, which is now consistent really sets the tone for the thought patterns that flow through my days.

The Carnivore way of eating has made a tremendous impact in my area of anxiety. Now when faced with otherwise large challenges I rarely get overwhelmed and often feel excellent moving through them.

My energy and my sleep have all made exceptional leaps in improvements. My mental focus and lack of distraction from gut and anxiety issues is now better than it has ever been. My skin has cleared up and I often receive comments on how clear it is.

The "Superfoods"

As I mentioned earlier I'd been following influencers in the health space; specifically Dave Asprey and Rhonda Patrick. Both promote different "Superfoods": Asprey with Coffee, Patrick, smoothies. Prior to Carnivore, I had the best coffee and best superfood smoothies!

My smoothies were loaded with "Superfoods": kale, spinach, almond butter, blueberries, flax seed, chia seeds, local fresh honey, cocoa nibs: naked whey protein - what I believed to be the ultimate mix. This daily combination of these coffees and smoothies were major triggers for my anxiety. The Carnivore Diet eliminated all of that. Once I was able to wean myself off these items and allow my body to heal the results were incredible.

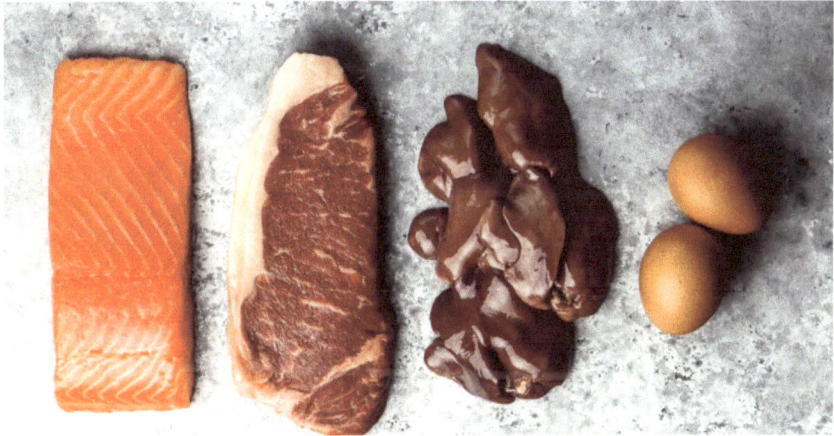

Image: Varying Carnivore foods

—— 4. THE CARNIVORE DIET ——
WHAT IS IT, AND WHY?

The Carnivore Diet is a diet constructed purely of animal foods. It is the complete removal of all plant molecules. It is kind of similar to the Whole30 Diet in that you are eliminating certain foods from your diet to see how your body responds. But on the Carnivore Diet there are absolutely no vegetables or fruits.

It is a powerful elimination diet that is showing huge promise in the treatment of a slew of disorders and disease. People thrive by removing potentially triggering foods from their diet, while zeroing in on the highest, most nutrient dense foods available.

Some of the success stories we see in the carnivore community revolve around treatments of long-standing: addiction, allergies, arthritis, asthma, anxiety, autoimmune, back pain, cardiovascular, dental, digestion, diabetes, weight loss, joint pain, mood, mental health, psoriasis, respiratory, skin, sleep, hormones and fatigue.

So why would one want to embark on this diet?

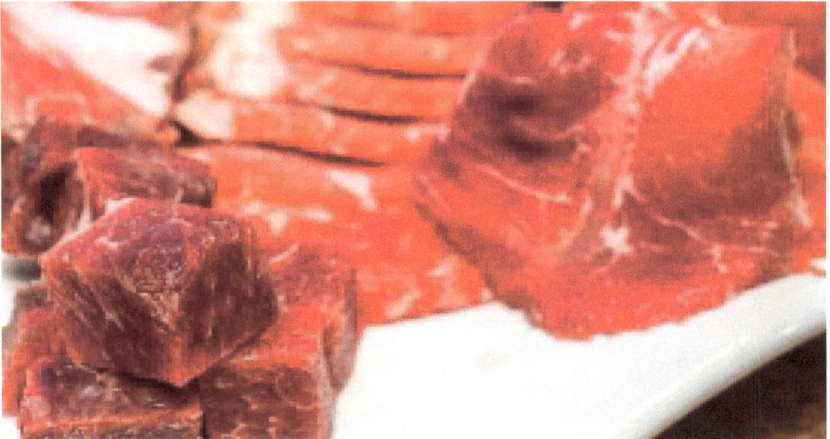

Image:freepik.com

A. Many Plants are Toxic

The Carnivore Diet is a powerful, nutrient rich, low inflammatory, low immune triggering elimination diet. Very few people react negatively to high quality grass fed beef.

Plants don't want to be eaten and cannot run from their predators. They've co-evolved with animals over millions of years and created natural toxins as their defense mechanism to kill off and limit predation. Molecules such as: glutens, lectins, polyphenols, sulforaphane, resveratrol, goitrogens, carotenoids are natural pesticides created by plants to fend off predators.

"Superfoodists" and brands selling these plant-based products have largely focused on the benefits highlighting aspects of studies and literature showing **only the benefits** to consuming them as humans.

When you look at studies on the entirety of the mechanism of which these molecules impact the human we see a very different picture. Polyphenols can tear gut lining, sulforaphane disrupts precursors that create adequate thyroid hormone, resveratrol can damage DNA There's a much different and darker picture around the entire impact and

consumption of these molecules that we're just now starting to understand and see.

Many argue these are xeno hermetic and antioxidative, meaning, they function a lot like exercise in stressing your system, but not too much, allowing you to bounce back stronger. But *unlike exercise or environmental stress, many plant molecules create collateral damage beyond the targeted stress that leads to a net negative effect on the human body.* Damage the human body struggles to bounce back from, especially with the constant bombardment of molecules continually attacking our bodies.

This can result in chronic disease, sometimes very quickly, other times over periods of months or even years.

The idea of consuming foods that trigger the human body antioxidant pathways, molecules that were designed to kill off insects and other predators, may be more harmful than healthful. Let's take a look further at some of these compounds and how they impact the human body.

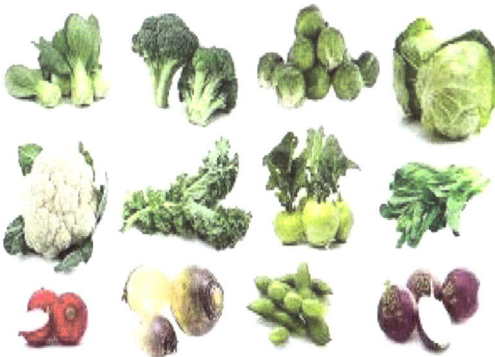

Image: Potentially damaging cruciferous vegetables

Keep in mind cooking, preparation and the sourcing time (whether it was ripe or not) can all have a dramatic impact on the "toxic" load of the plant molecules outlined here.

Goitrogens

These are a class of substances that are goitrogenic. Goitrogens compete with iodine uptake at the thyroid level and can contribute to hypothyroidism (reduced thyroid). Cruciferous vegetables can be quite goitrogenic. Many are hailed as excellent in health, but not actually be the case. That's right, the broccoli your mom told you to finish may in fact be limiting your thyroid production and lowering your overall energy levels.

Saponins

Another class of compounds found in licorice, legumes (the pea family), quinoa and spinach, as well as other plants, is a compound called saponin. It is a bitter-tasting compound that evolved as a defense system that can block nutrient absorption, damage metabolism and kill cells. Specifically, saponins are known to disrupt fat metabolism, increase intestinal permeability (break your gut lining), cleave cholesterol (alter the molecular form in an unnatural way), disrupt endocrine function and are generally toxic to our cells. There are many more classes of plant molecules that, although marketed as extremely healthy, can create collateral damage in the human body.

Gluten

Today's gluten found in wheat, rye and barley is a sticky protein known to damage the gut lining. This leads to a whole slew of health issues from acne to diabetes to cancer.

Lectins

Popularized by Dr. Steven Gundry, lectins are found in grains, legumes and plant seeds. They are known to cause gut damage which can lead to autoimmune response and inflammation.

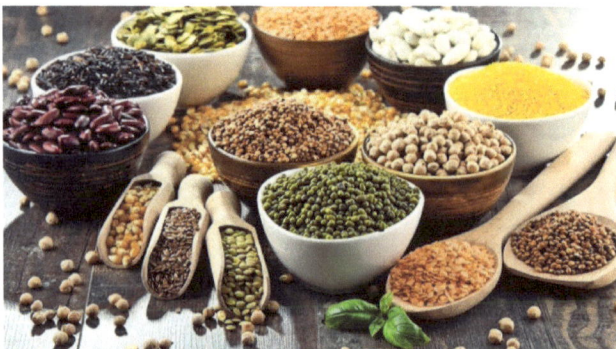
Image: Saponins

Oxalates

Found in higher concentrations in "superfoods" such as spinach, kale and cacao powder. Oxalates bind to calcium in your body and can accumulate in the thyroid as well as kidneys. This can strip mineral absorption and lead to health complications such as kidney stones and hypothyroidism. Roughly 80% of kidney stones are linked to oxalate formation. [50]

Phytic Acid

Found in seeds, nuts and beans. Phytic Acid reduces absorption of specific minerals from foods and strips the body of absorbing valuable minerals. It's known to chelate (bind) to certain essential minerals: calcium, iron, zinc and magnesium, reducing your body's ability to absorb them. Human guts can produce an enzyme phytase to help break it down, but it's not well known how effective we are at it.

Sulforaphane

Famously echoed as a cancer-curing messiah by Rhonda Patrick, Sulforaphane is found in cruciferous rich foods. Think broccoli, broccoli sprouts, brussel sprouts, bok choy, and cabbage. Sulforaphane in these plants is innately toxic to animal cells, destroying membranes and mitochondria. Promoted for its cancer-killing properties, sadly it doesn't discriminate and, a lot

like chemotherapy, destroys healthy cells as well.

Polyphenols

Dave Asprey's favorite superfood to coffee is known to break gut lining, cause leaky gut and a number of health problems related to that. [52] [53]

Resveratrol

Another favorite among the supplement industry for its longevity benefits. Resveratrol is also a phenol produced by plants under attack. Resveratrol is found in grapes, berries and nuts. And you guessed it, it also damages our gut barrier.

NRF2-Pathway

Much of the benefits of the molecules discussed hinge on the hermetic effect and more specifically the activation of our liver's natural antioxidant producing NRF2 pathway. Yes it's true the NRF2 pathway is a potent way of introducing antioxidants into the body. Generally it is great for our bodies to have antioxidants in them. But how those antioxidants are being triggered matters.

Did you know ingesting poison will trigger your NRF2 pathway? That's right, drinking alcohol and smoking will activate this pathway. But we wouldn't indulge in those activities to boost our glutathione production (a natural antioxidant produced) because we realize their collateral effects would far outweigh the benefits of this excess antioxidant produced in response. We realize in these cases there's a very clear and acute, often punctuated affect on the body that is a net negative.

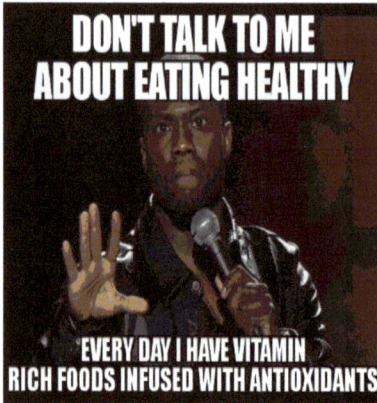

DON'T TALK TO ME ABOUT EATING HEALTHY

EVERY DAY I HAVE VITAMIN RICH FOODS INFUSED WITH ANTIOXIDANTS

Image: "Healthy" foods meme

Eating foods that are "antioxidant" purely for gaining "antioxidants" is all the rave in the health food industry. But what if we instead focused on reducing oxidation and consuming a diet low in creating that oxidation and rich in all the essential nutrients all while limiting plant toxicity? (Hint - Carnivore)

With many other plant molecules we believe we may be seeing a similar situation. Their benefits are outweighed by their collateral damage. Though we may not feel the impact as intensely or abruptly as drinking or smoking long-forming nutrient deficiencies, hormone imbalances, leaky gut and damage to other parts of the body can occur.

B.Treatment of long standing disease/disorders

In the carnivore community people are seeing real success and reversal of serious issues. It's still early and these stories are anecdotes but the results in the community are powerful, and show a real story of just how impactful the diet is.

I. Lose Weight, Gain Muscles, Improve Vitality.

The Carnivore Diet gives your body the building blocks it needs to improve hormone production. Weight-loss is largely a hormone game. Eating at a deficit is a piece of it, but you must have optimal hormones or the body won't "burn" excess fat.

II. Blood Sugar

Blood sugar must be tightly regulated in order to avoid damaging vessels, vital organs and your nervous system among other things. Our bodies are very much biochemical systems. Insulin is the primary hormone your body releases in order to do this.

Insulin tells your body's fat cells to store the excess glucose from the carbohydrates. Fat cells open up and receive this energy.

When insulin is flowing and signaling to your cells it's impossible for them to release and "burn" their energy reserves. The cells are being told to store, not burn.

When insulin is low, you can utilize those energy stores and actually burn fat from your stores.

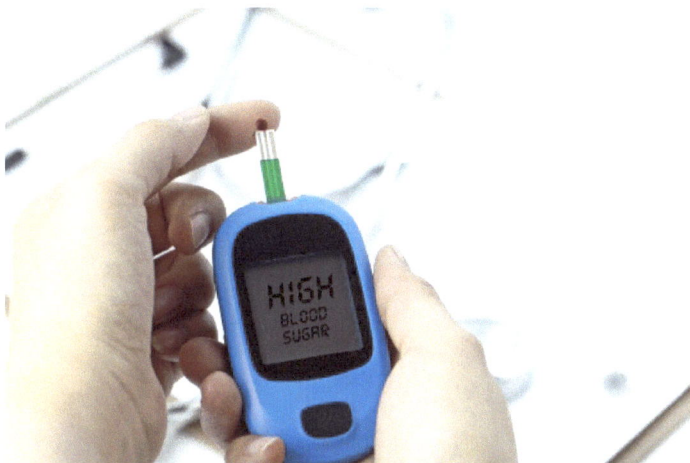

Image: freepik.com

Most chronic disease is likely related to chronically elevated levels of insulin. Anytime you have elevated hormones in the body receptors can down-regulate their sensitivity. And many people become insulin resistant. Alzheimer's has actually been referred to as type III diabetes [1]. We'll talk about weight loss in more detail in a later section.

III. Reduce Allergies

Allergies are the result of histamine building up in the body. It's a natural process of fighting off foreign molecules the body finds harmful. Foods are one of the biggest sources of allergies. We'll learn how a properly formulated fresh food Carnivore Diet can help treat this. Bonus, some Carnivore foods can actually help naturally break down excess histamine build up. There's a specific section all about this.

IV. Improvement in Mood, Depression, Anxiety

I shared some of my personal stories of anxiety, depression and panic. This was the hardest time in my life and I often felt alone and stuck with a life sentence of disorder.

Mental illness is painful and isolating because it's very hard for others to understand, unless they experienced the same pain.

There were points when I thought I was literally crazy. Bouts of anxiety ridden insomnia that left me feeling very disturbed and stuck. I can safely say this is no longer the case. I am quite certain this diet has made an equal, if not greater, impact on this area of my life, in spite of all the counseling and self discovery.

Countless anecdotes from the Carnivore community, mine included, have testified to the substantial improvements in mood and mental health. The Carnivore Diet ensures the brain gets unique required nutrients ONLY found in animal foods to properly function: B12, DHA, EPA fatty acids.

Hormones play a critical role in how you feel. Carnivore Diets are rich in quality proteins and fats which help your liver produce the dozen egg yolks or so worth of cholesterol you need everyday. Sugar and carbohydrates have been shown to negatively impact this.

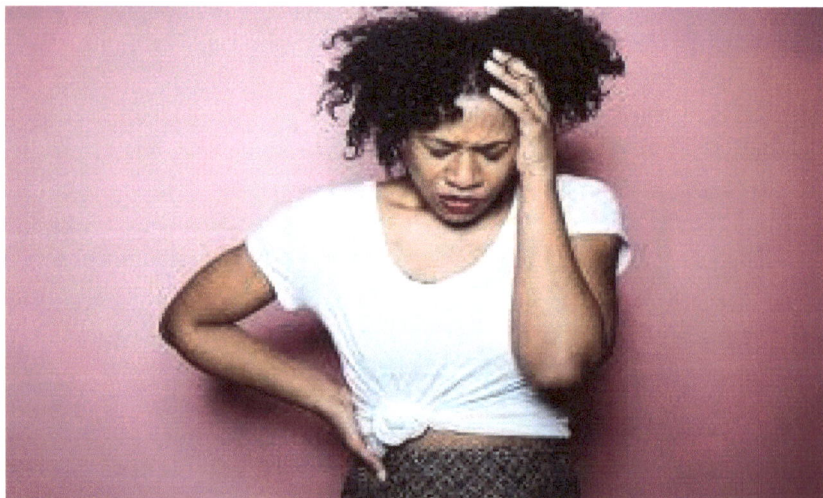
Image: Gut issues

Iron, Serotonin and Dopamine

Animal iron (heme) is much more absorbable for humans. Absorbed at a rate of 15-35% while plant iron is only ~2-20%. It is estimated that roughly 5% of vegans are iron deficient (ancmic). Iron is a cofactor enzyme that is 2responsible for dopamine (motivation) and serotonin (feel good) synthesis. These are the major molecules we believe can support mental health.

Chris Palmer MD assistant professor of Psychiatry at Harvard and practicing psychiatrist at McClean [45] - (the hospital my very own grandmother attended) is currently doing tremendous work with ketogenic and Carnivore Diets to treat his patients. In some cases reversing long-standing (once thought of as) severe mental illness cases that would be life-long sentences.

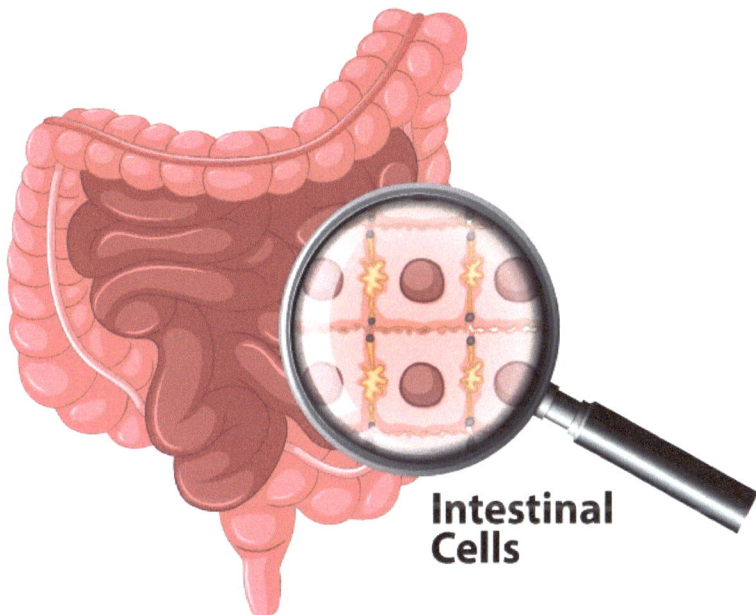

Intestinal Cells

C. Gut Issues

This has always, even with Carnivore been an issue for me, I've had to learn how to do the Carnivore Diet in a certain way - as I'll teach you in this book to properly manage this. Like many, I thought more fiber would help - but it was actually the removal of fiber that helped me see improvement. That in combination with less inflammation, and the removal of plant molecules that can increase gut permeability (breakage) has led to tremendous relief and ease. Mental clarity and a much reduced anxious state have also been a by-product. Whenever I deviate from my diet I am almost immediately am reminded through feelings within my gut.

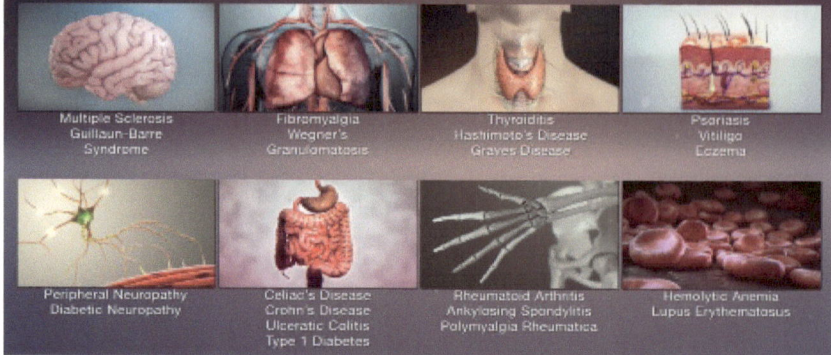

https://www.scientificanimations.com/autoimmune-diseases-symptoms-and-treatments/

D. Autoimmune Disease/Disorders

These are a class of diseases defined by the body attacking healthy cells. Arthritis, Lupus, Celiac, MS and Type 1 Diabetes are all considered in this class. *The Carnivore Diet helps with many of these conditions by restricting the foods that trigger inflammation and autoimmune signaling.* When the body isn't constantly bombarded with foods putting it on high alert, and damage for an extended period of time we see symptoms subside and often go into remission. Unfortunately many of these foods have been categorized as "healthy."

E. Energy, Cognitive Function

Ketone bodies have been shown to be more beneficial to mental performance and overall stable mental energy. They are metabolically more efficient providing more energy per unit oxygen and less reactive oxygen species. That said, when I first tried "Keto" I found a lot of challenges with maintaining gut health. All the oils, rendered, condensed oil fats and butters, did not sit well with me. Bacon and avocados didn't do well with me. You will see they have their own problems.

The gut has 100M neurons. By moving over to an animal-based diet I was able to really improve how I felt from a gut perspective while remaining ketogenic. This has been an absolute game-changer in terms of being able to sustain this way of eating. The mental performance has been incredible.

Okay so now that we've gone over a few of the reasons, let's dive into the anthropological thinking around Carnivore.

— 5. ANCESTRAL ALIGNMENT —
AND THE BIOCHEMISTRY

One of the greatest hypotheses for why we're seeing such powerful results within the Carnivore community is the idea of how well it is ancestrally aligned with our bodies and what they're intended to consume nutritionally.

Humans evolved from primates ~ 15-20M years ago. As we evolved several major changes have been observed from records indicating what happened.

- At first we were simply land dwellers spending more time on the ground and more time erect and upright.

- Around 2.6M years ago something unique happened. Our brains started growing rapidly in size as a species.

- Our guts shrunk in size, the colon and intestinal tract became significantly smaller.

- Our guts became highly acidic - in many cases PH levels down in the 1.5-2 range are recorded in humans now.

- Our shoulders adapted to throwing vs hanging.

- Our limbs and bodies became longer and leaner supporting faster and more agile ground movement. Also supporting seeing higher and further across lands.

- Fossil records indicate that we started using tools.

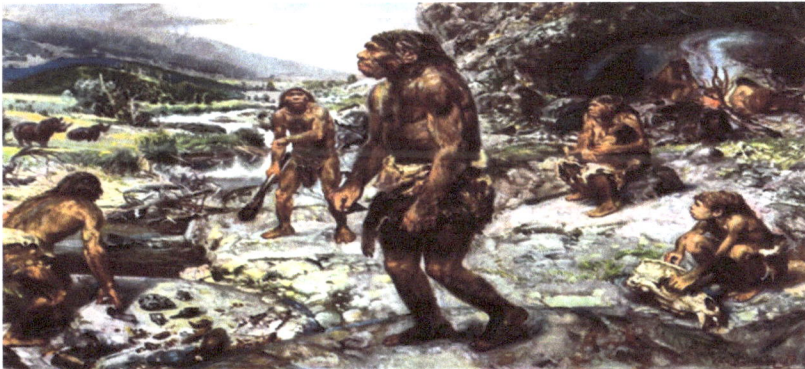

Image: Prehistoric man

Why did this all happen? One major argument is that we experienced a cooling of the environment and plants became much more scarce.

Around 2.6M years ago we saw the current Ice Age [2] - Quaternary period, we're currently still in and nearing the tail end of the 5th ice age. Our early ancestors - Homo Habilis were stuck in a very unique period.

Plant foods are largely seasonal and are much less abundant in cooler climates. As the ice age began cooling the climate plants died off and the food types these early homo species could source shifted to those from animals.

Animal foods provide a high calorie per volume and as these early ancestors started consuming more of these foods, they're biology shifted.

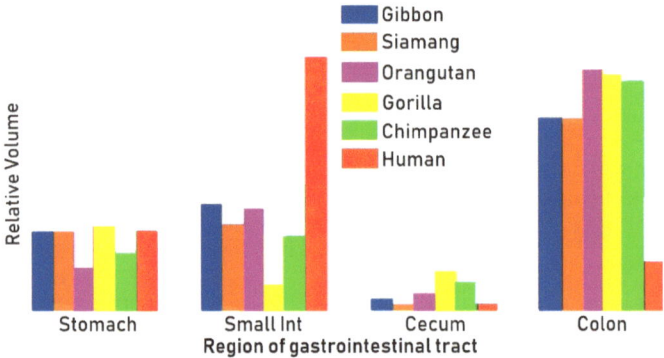

Image source: Researchgate.net - University of Melbourne, David Bravo

Changes in Gut

Where our primate ancestors needed long guts to ferment large amounts of fiber into fats, our new diet required that our guts become much more acidic. Primates and other herbivores have a gut pH in the range of 4-5 while carnivorous felines and canines typically have a pH of 2-3, while homo sapiens often get to 1.3-1.5.

The high acidity of our stomachs is metabolically expensive to sustain and is unlikely to occur by accident. It evolved to handle the flesh and remains that contained pathogens and bacteria the acid could kill off. It also helped break down dietary protein more efficiently than with lower pH levels.

Records show that these early Homo species started using tools. These tools were used to crack open the bones of carcuses and left over remains of animals their predators couldn't get into. Bones and skulls containing marrow and brains rich in fat and proteins became a staple of a food source for this early homo species.

The two most metabolically expensive systems in the animal body are the digestive system and the brain. For humans, the brain accounts for only ~ 2-3% of the body mass but uses 20% of the metabolic energy.

Over hundreds of thousands of years enterprising homo species body's continued to adapt to the cooling climate and more nutrient dense animal food sources. At the same time, several of the large megafauna (wholly mammouths) animals and their remains became more and more scarce as their plant food became scarcer.[3]

We could no longer pillage leftover remains from these animals and had to adapt to hunting smaller, more agile animals. The shoulders and limbs shifted from being optimized for hanging amongst trees to supporting the throwing of objects and agile erect ground moving to track hunting animals. Being able to stand allowed us to scour grasslands and track our prey more effectively.

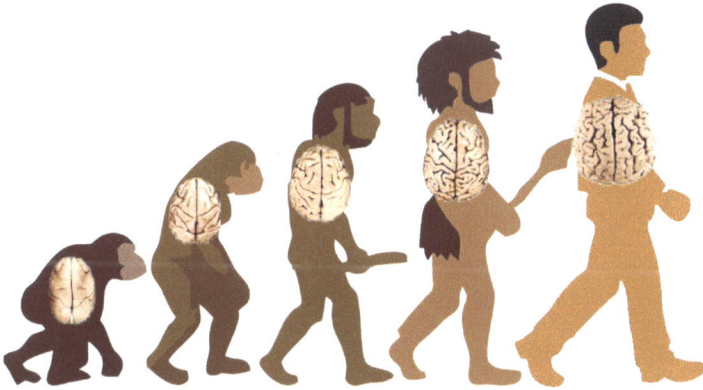

ARM POSITIONS DURING THROWING

Chimp

Chimpanzees throw very poorly, despite being incredibly strong and athletic

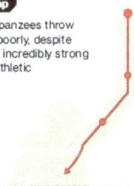

Human

One of the evolutionary changes is the ability to twist the upper arm bone

Chimp

Adult male chimps can only throw objects at about **20mph**, one-third of the speed of a 12-year-old child who is a good thrower

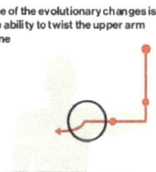

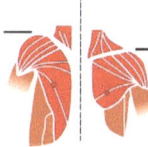

Human

Human shoulders are at a lower position on the torso which efficiently utilises the energy stored in the tendons and ligaments

Image Source: University of Washington

Some researchers suggest our evolution of shoulders was one of the greatest advancements that enabled us to evolve to the top of the food chain. [46]

What About Our Teeth?!

A major argument around the biology of humans and why we are intended to eat primarily plant foods is our dental design. We humans lack the abundance of sharp incisors and canines - used to tear and shred animal flesh prevalent in many other carnivorous animals.

Carnivore Teeth   Herbivore

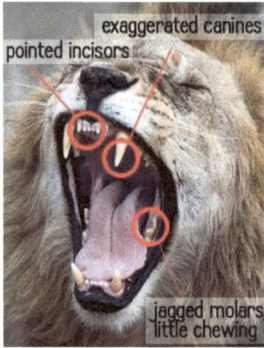
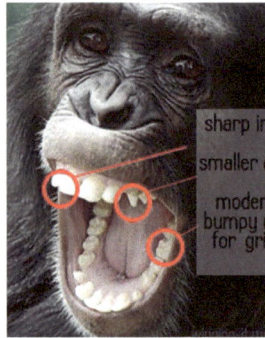
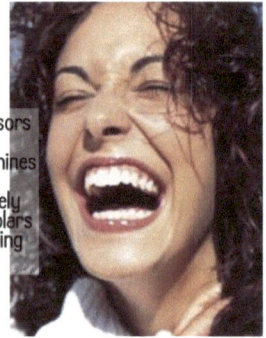

Image: Teeth comparison feline, primate, human

But evolution is powered by necessity. When we look at fossil records we see early homo species used tools. [4] Specifically sharp edges and rocks being used. These tools gave early hominids a tremendous advantage as we were able to crack, tear, and break into hard to reach places even carnivores and their teeth couldn't get into. Our hands evolved as it became advantageous to have more agility and dexterity to handle tools with these parts of our limbs and **the necessity of incisors and teeth to shred animal foods never existed.**

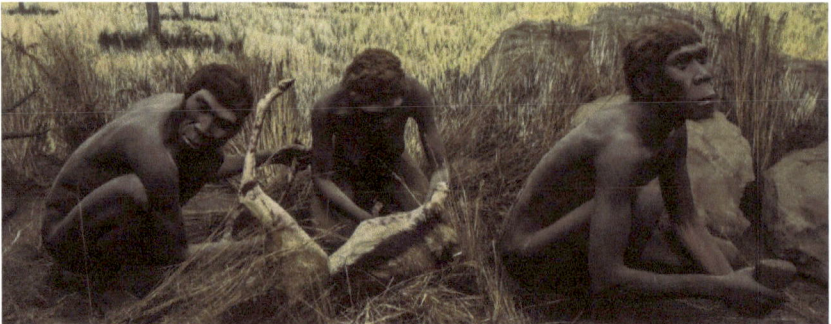

Image. Prehistoric homo species

A large hypothesis for how we grew such large human brains was our new diet rich in fatty acids and cholesterol, all primary ingredients that make up and are required by the human brain. That new diet of animal foods, requiring a smaller but more acidic gut fueled our evolution.

During this time frame of 2.5 million years we saw the largest brain sizes evolve, going from 400cc -> 1500cc (Neaderthals, 40,000 years ago) then back down to current homo sapiens 1350ccs. Fossils of these ancestors have been discovered showing their skull sizes.

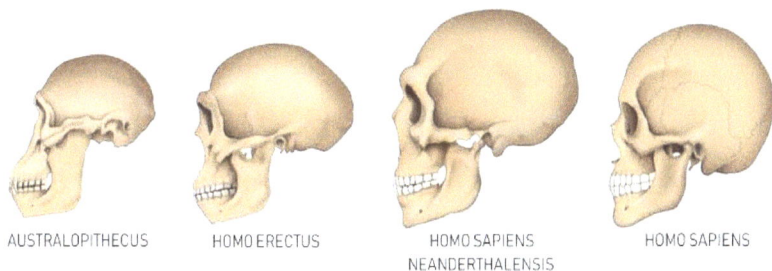

AUSTRALOPITHECUS   HOMO ERECTUS   HOMO SAPIENS NEANDERTHALENSIS   HOMO SAPIENS

Image: Skull evolution into homo sapiens

Additionally *it should be stated that the vast majority of plant foods available in the human diet today were not present in nature, both in their form, and in their quantity.* Many of today's common plant foods have been genetically modified [5] to improve yield, taste and survive the onslaught of predators that would otherwise decimate them.

I actually think GMO cropping was a good thing for the planet and our species - if you read The Rational Optimist by Matt Ridley, his perspective is one of the best I've heard on this. It has allowed humans to innovate and produce greater yields of plants at a much higher efficiency to feed people. That said, the context here is more about ancestral alignment, and if it is what is most optimal for our biology.

The majority of fruit today is shipped in from 1,000s of miles across the world. It never would've been available year round for consumption outside rare equatorial regions.

In nature we see almost no cases outside milk where there is a combination of fat and sugar. And we almost never see processed refined carbs like sugar. Societies do exist with high carb [6] consumption - tubers in particular seem to be the staple for these - and still thrive without cases of heart disease, obesity and the chronic western diseases we see.

That said, if you went outdoors today and were forced to survive as a vegetarian - you would most certainly struggle and quickly fade away. The tree leaves, grass, and bark would overload your gut with fiber, with almost no calories or protein. If you were lucky enough to stumble across a corn field (which would not be natural) you might do well until you develop diabetes from the constant elevated insulin due to it's unnatural higher glycemic load.

But perhaps you're a lucky homo sapien born somewhere warm or tropical with coconuts or avocados - surviving on those items alone would lead to serious protein and nutrient deficiencies. You'd have to find fish and animals and learn to hunt and scavenge in order to provide proper nutrition for your body.

Humans evolved as facultative carnivores, who could eat some plant foods in times of famine alongside animal foods. Our brains, guts, limbs and what makes us human-beings able to read this book, the ability to think cognitively, is largely a result of our evolution of consuming animal foods.

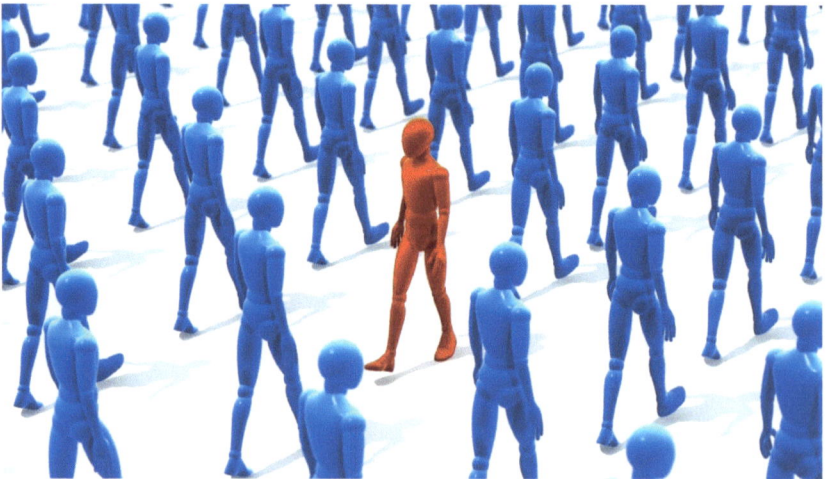

Image: Heading in the opposite direction of the group

Defying "Conventional" Health Advice

When I first started learning about a keto diet four years ago I was worried about my heart health. Heart disease runs in my family and almost everything I could find online as well as my conventional MD suggested a diet rich in saturated fat and cholesterol was surely going to severely increase my risk for heart disease.

For about 2-3 months I had serious moments of anxiety as I continued to eat a high fat "toxic" "damaging" diet. That anxiety lead to more discomfort and doubt around the diet. I desperately looked for literature to betterunderstand and educate myself. All the eggs, avocados, bacon, cheese, almonds I was taking in was putting me in ketosis and making for very clear thinking but I was genuinely concerned it could impact me negatively longer term.

As I persisted and noticed improved energy levels and found more articles and books (Mercola, Sisson, Ferris and Asprey) promoting these ways of eating, I gained confidence that what I was doing wasn't hurting me but was actually the best thing for me. My anxiety around the diet subsided and I started experiencing the benefits.

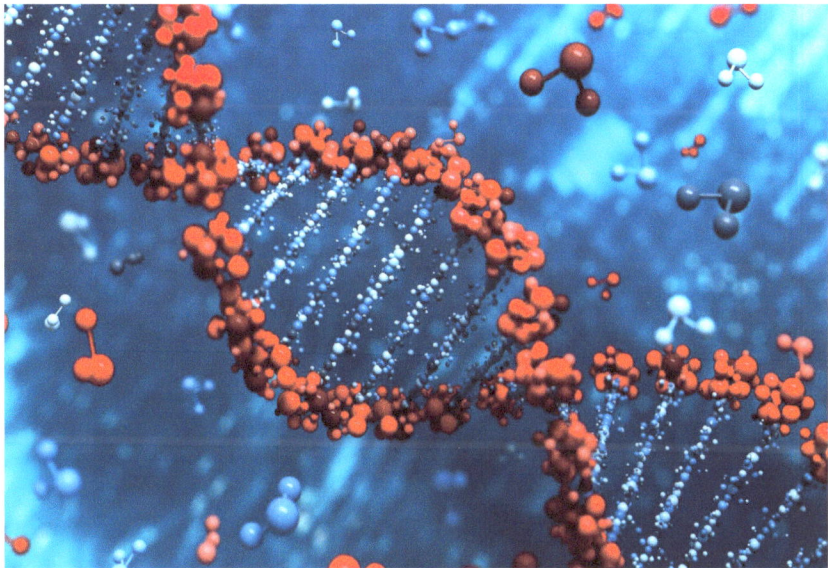

Image: DNA Helix, Molecules

Biochemistry:

I realize anthropology is subject to interpretation and much can be conjecture. But I do believe more than anything the biochemistry of animal foods shows a very powerful and compelling story of why they are the primary form of foods humans are intended to consume.

Back in the 1970s researchers such as Ancel Keys led many to believe that animal foods, specifically saturated fats and LDL cholesterol they elevated were damaging to human cardiovascular systems. In his famous Seven Countries Study (SCS) that attempted to show consuming red meat leads to obesity, carcinogenic molecules and hurts humans, **he intentionally left out** populations that clearly contradicted his hypotheses. [7]

When you break down the fundamental nutrients the human body needs, what you find is that the "essential," meaning *the nutrients we must get from foods - largely come from animal foods.* The essential nutrients plants provide are much less bioavailable and often need a conversion within the human body.

Additionally there are clear antinutrients [8] absent in animal foods that plants contain that inhibit mineral absorption, impact hormone function and impact our bodies in a number of other negative ways. Oxalates in spinach and Kale bind to calcium, iron and magnesium. [9] Phytic acid present in many plant foods binds to iron, zinc, manganese and copper. "Superfoods" like kale, collard greens, and brussel sprouts all cause thyroid swelling.

Essential Nutrients of Life

13 Vitamins	18 Minerals	10 Amino Acids
Vitamin A	Calcium	Histidine
Vitamin D	Chlorine	Isoleucine
Vitamin E	Chromium	Leucine
Vitamin K (Potassium)	Cobalt	Lysine
Thiamine (B1)	Copper	Methoinine
Riboflavin (B2)	Iodine +	Nonessential Nitrogen
Niacin (B3)	Iron	Phenylalanine
Biotin	Magnesium	Theonine
Panthothenic Acid (B5)	Manganese	Tryptophan
Vitamin B6	Molybdenum	Valine
Vitamin B12	Phosporus	
Folic Acid	Selenium	**1 Protein**
Vitamin C	Silicon	
	Sodium	**1 Water**
1 Carbohydrate	Sulfur	
Glucose	Tin	
	Vanadium	
1 Fat (lipid)	Zinc	**TOTAL = 45**
Linoleic Acid		

**Your body can make whatever else it needs
from these 45 essential nutrients.**

https://steemit.com/health/@corpdetoxbliss/optimum-health-are-we-treating-the-symptoms-or-the-cause

There are 45 essential nutrients the human body needs that must be obtained from the environment. These nutrients cannot be produced from within. Some can be converted from certain sources but this list shows them. [56]

Omega 3 vs Omega 6 Fats:

The human body needs omega-3 fatty acids. Benefits [10] include fighting depression, improving brain and eye health, and reducing inflammation. And there's quite a few more. Although omega-6 (Ω) fats are important to humans, balance is key. Some studies go as far as to suggest a balance of 1:1 Ω-6:Ω-3 ratio. [11] That said 25% of your fats in Ω-3 form (4:1 ratio) seems to be sufficient for a majority of the health benefits.

With the fear around red meat, dietary cholesterol and saturated fat, plant seed oils have become a major component of human diets in the last several decades. These oils are highly processed and are almost exclusively omega-6 in their fatty acid profile. A diet favoring these throws the optimal ratio totally out of whack for optimal human health. Many studies

suggest modern Western diets now climb to ratios north of 15 times as much omega-6 as omega-3 ratios - contributing to high inflammation and disease. [12]

DHA & EPA vs ALA:

The animal forms of omega-3 fats are DHA or EPA and there is only a small portion found in plants; ALA. You may have heard of some of these plant "superfoods" flax and chia seeds. But the reality is that humans can only convert between 0.5-9%[13] of ALA into EPA and DHA.

From studies it seems women in their fertile years have a unique ability to convert at a higher rate - up to x2 that of young men - but still likely insufficient - this may have to do with the importance of DHA in the development of their baby.

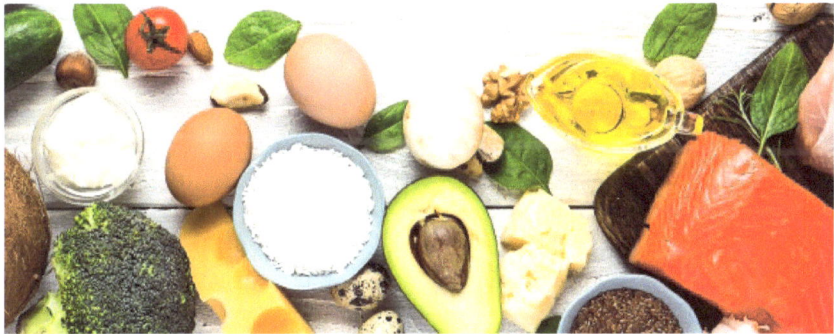

image: freepik.com

Vitamin A:

Critical to skin, eye and nerve health. Protects cells from free radical damage and powers our immune systems. Animal form is retinol, plant form is beta-carotene. Studies suggest the human body converts plant form anywhere from 4:1 -> 28:1, depending on the plant form. [14]

Iron -> Heme Iron:

Iron is essential in the body for transporting oxygen from the lungs through the blood to your cells. Hemoglobin represents 2/3s of the iron in the body. Heme iron is the form humans need which is found ONLY in animal foods, iron found in plant foods is poorly absorbed and one reason why iron deficiencies are extremely common amongst vegans.

I carry a genetic polymorphism for absorbing high levels of iron. In my last round of labs I had elevated ferritin levels over the reference range. [15] Ancestrally we probably lost blood from time to time to reduce these stores from bleeding and other environmental stressors less prevalent now. In my case I simply plan on giving blood 2-3x/year.

D2 -> D3:

I did a whole video on this topic here. Vitamin D3, is technically not even a vitamin, it's actually classified as a prohormone [16]. Plants only provide vitamin D2, your body must convert it. Vitamin D3, the form your body needs is found in moderate amounts in animal foods but really is mostly obtained indirectly through ultraviolet B light radiation reaching the skin. Roughly 90% is produced through this process.

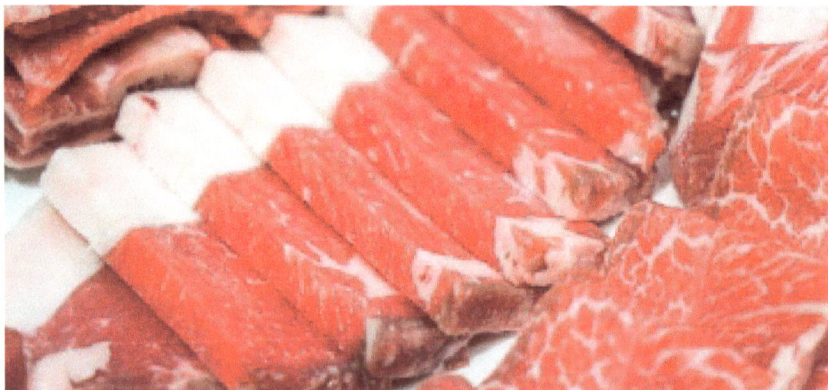

Image: freepik.com

I believe so strongly in the importance of this and other impacts that affect us with respect to light that I have written a book on the topic of light.

Vitamin K1 vs K2:

K2 has a remarkable ability to cure nutrient deficiencies and degenerative disease. It's regarded as a critical nutrient for many of the body's needs - organ, bone, brain and kidney health are just a few. K2 is the form your body needs, animal foods (egg yolks and dark chicken) are some of the best sources of K2. Your body can utilize fat to convert plant form K1 into K2, but plants do not provide the form you need.

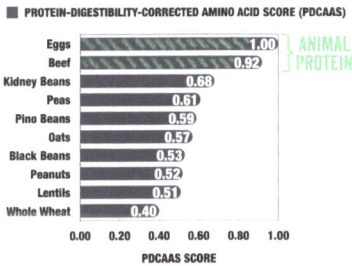

PROTEIN-DIGESTIBILITY-CORRECTED AMINO ACID SCORE (PDCAAS)

Food	PDCAAS Score
Eggs	1.00
Beef	0.92
Kidney Beans	0.68
Peas	0.61
Pino Beans	0.59
Oats	0.57
Black Beans	0.53
Peanuts	0.52
Lentils	0.51
Whole Wheat	0.40

ANIMAL PROTEIN

PDCAAS SCORE

Image: PDCAAS score given to foods for protein digestibility and absorbability

Essential Amino Acids:

The building blocks of the human body's muscles. Animal foods contain these in complete form, typically containing all of them. Plant proteins struggle to meet these requirements. In fact we've created a very specific score that accounts for their digestibility called the protein digestibility, corrected amino acid score (PDCAA). Synthetically created pea and soy proteins (which comes with a whole slew of health concerns) come close, but Whey, Egg, Milk, Cheese, Chicken, Fish and Beef are all more complete, more absorbable forms.

"Animal foods contain these in complete form, typically containing all of them. Plant proteins struggle to meet these requirements."

Folate:

Known as vitamin B9 it is necessary for cell growth and metabolism. Carriers of the common MTHFR gene variants - have trouble creating the MTHFR enzyme that converts dietary folate from plants into the animal form L-methylfolate - which is critical in neurotransmitter synthesis. Anywhere from **15-25% of the population** can be a carrier of this. Though it's present in plant foods in varying amounts - **beef liver is by far the best source for this**. Plant foods such as asparagus, broccoli, spinach and broccoli sprouts contain some folate but they also pack (as we've discussed earlier) a slew of other anti-nutrients and potentially damaging molecules.

Side note - Nutritionists have fortified many processed foods with its synthetic form of vitamin B9, Folic acid. It's very hard to overdo folate but people who supplement folic acid can experience negative effects. It can hide signs of B12 deficiency and lead to nerve damage. [57]

— 6. ERRORS IN STUDIES FOR — CONCERN

Epidemiology (literal Greek for "the study of what is upon people") is the modern approach often taken to studying and determining distribution patterns in society of health and disease conditions within a defined population. Think epidemic, now defining disease or disorders within populations.

Historically this has been researcher's and scientist's way to identify problems within a subset of people and look further into potential causal relationships. First we see a group of people, then we see a disease. We then look at the habits and patterns that might be linked. This makes a lot of sense. Initially we are likely to see a correlation among a large population which would then direct our attention towards digging further and studying more closely to research

That said, we must always be careful - what we look for we will often find. If you're searching for a particular relationship or link, then you're much more likely to "discover" evidence and information that supports that hypothesis. In fact there's a scientific term for this exact phenomenon called "Confirmation Bias." This is a very real bias researchers have.

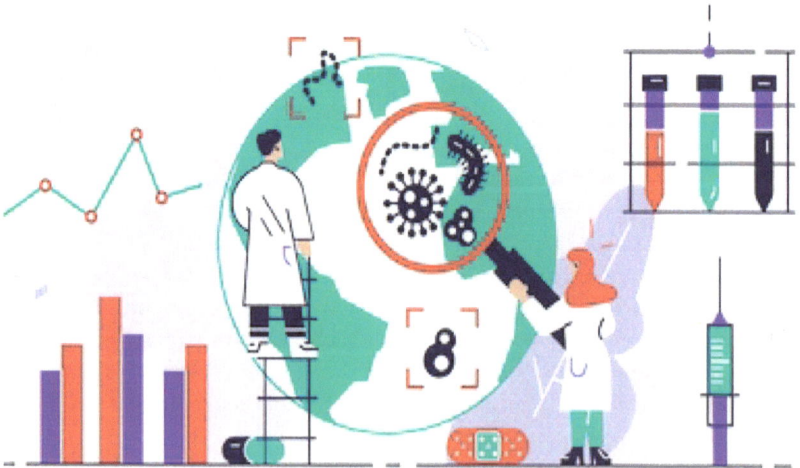

Image: Researchers around the world

Ancel Keys, the "father" of the lipid hypothesis who famously conducted the Seven Countries Study brought mainstream public, the fear of saturated fat. This led to fears of high cholesterol, terrifying Americans that saturated fats were causes for heart disease. When we actually look at Ancel Key's data, he intentionally left out contradicting countries where people eat a lot of fat but have little heart disease, such as Holland and Norway. As well as countries where fat consumption is low but the rate of heart disease is high, such as Chile.

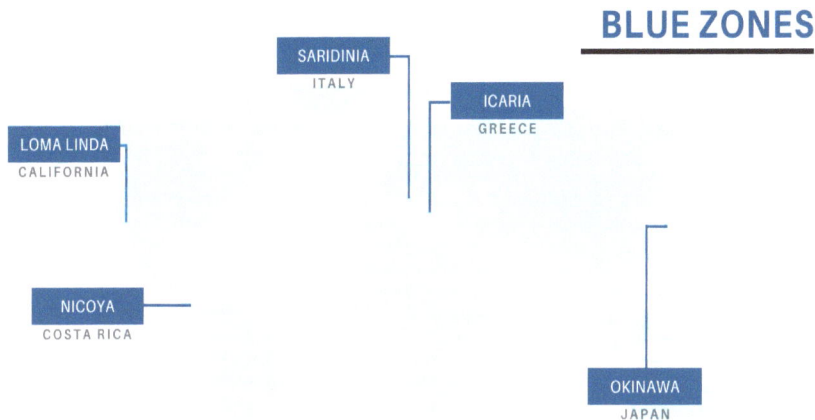

Image: Regions of the world labeled "The Blue Zones"

The Blue Zones

The Blue Zones are regions of the world claimed to include populations that live longer than average life expectancies. They are often referred to in epidemiology as having exceptional health. The exact regions are Loma Linda, California the Nicoya peninsula in Costa Rica, Sardinia, Italy, Icaria, Greece and Okinawa, a southern Japanese island; the five officially recognized blue zones.

Loma Linda California white males live on average 7 years longer than the average white male in California. Sardinian males in Italy live to 80 while the average American male to 77

Many argue that a major contributing factor to the longevity of the populations within these regions is their emphasis on plant-based diets. But there are significant lifestyle factors that have not been controlled in this argument. I'd argue these are likely much more the reason for their superior health and longevity.

These populations tend to get significantly more sunshine, outdoor activity, social and emotional support from their communities. We know sunlight [17], movement and exercise all contribute immensely to overall health and longevity. There are several studies that show a sedentary lifestyle with activities such as TV watching directly correlates with shorter life expectancy. [18]

When looking at the Blue zones, several arguments don't hold well. For example the people of Okinawa were notorious for eating pork and much less rice than other regions in Asia. Okinawans also have the lowest life expectancy of the major Japanese regions, all of which consume more meat.

Hong Kong and Singapore, countries with even longer life expectancies than Okinawa both consume substantial amounts of animal foods. In fact, Hong Kong has the highest life expectancy in the world. They also consume more meat than any other industrialized society in the world [47]. They also rank among the top 5 countries in the world with the highest IQ.

Hong Kong now has the highest life expectancy in the world

Rank	Country	Consumption	Population	Per Capita
	World	57,240,000	7,158,000,000	12.25
1	Hong Kong	582,000	7,219,700	123.51
2	Argentina	2,700,000	42,669,500	96.95
3	Uruguay	175,000	3,286,314	81.59
4	Brazil	7,925,000	201,032,714	60.40
5	United States	11,172,000	317,916,000	53.84
6	Australia	760,000	23,460,484	49.64
7	Chile	455,000	15,116,435	46.12
8	Paraguay	192,000	6,783,374	43.37
9	Canada	970,000	35,344,962	42.05
10	Kazakhstan	416,000	17,207,000	37.04

Life expectancy at birth (years), UN World Population Prospects 2015

Rank	State/Territory	Overall	Male	Female
1	Hong Kong	83.74	80.91	86.58
2	Japan	83.31	80.00	86.49
3	Italy	82.84	80.27	85.23
4	Switzerland	82.66	80.43	84.74
5	Singapore	82.64	79.59	85.61
6	Iceland	82.30	80.73	83.84
7	Spain	82.28	79.42	85.05
8	Australia	82.10	79.93	84.28
9	Israel	82.07	80.18	83.82
10	Sweden	81.93	80.10	83.71

Image source: Shanghai.ist

Of course this doesn't prove that meat is the "cause" for this longevity or improvement - but it certainly brings into question the epidemiological "evidence" that plant-based eating is the reason for longevity.

India and Bangladesh, two of the highest plant-based diet countries rank as some of the lowest in the world for life expectancy. I realize poverty rates and their infant mortality are higher but in India that is primarily plant-based, their rates of cardiovascular disease (25% of deaths) diabetes and prediabetes (25%) are some of the highest on the planet. When we look at subsets of the population that consume animal foods we see their risk factors go down. In fact, this study [54] showed that women who ate meat 5 times / week suffer from lower rates of obesity, heart disease, and cancer while having lower rates of insulin resistance and inflammation than non-meat eaters.

Again why would we think eating meat is a variable that causes cardiovascular disease (CVD) if we see the opposite diets but significant CVD? Clearly it's complex and more research needs to be done.

"The thing I have noticed is when anecdotes and the data disagree, the anecdotes are usually right. There's something wrong with the way you are measuring it."
Jeff Bezos (CEO/Founder Amazon)

Today we see several other societies that contradict that plant-based = heart health & longevity claims.

The Masai in Africa eat a diet almost exclusively of milk, meat and blood. Two thirds of their diet is animal fat loaded with cholesterol and they have virtually zero heart disease. (I suspect, movement, sunshine along with their rich regimen of high quality animal foods is keeping them extremely healthy).

Another case is the French Paradox [19] where we see the French having some of the lowest rates of CVD among industrialized societies despite consuming a diet much higher in saturated fat, (all that delicious cheese, fondue, butter chaucherie, duck.) yum!

Needless to say, there are societies on both ends of the equation. Looking at epidemiology is useful in helping form a hypothesis, but a hypothesis is not a theory until it has been rigorously tested, vetted and proven from real interventional trials and studies. And therein lies the entirety of this conundrum. We don't have those to support plant-based eating is truly the cause of health and longevity.

What we have, if anything, is clear contradicting epidemiology labeling and attributing factors in defiance of the plant-based anti-animal food, heart disease propaganda.

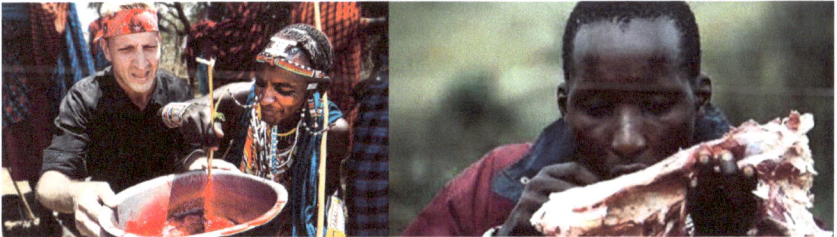

Image source: www.nation.co.ke

7. The TOXICITY OF RED MEAT
TMAO, mTOR, Neu5GC and Cancer

If you can't tell, I really did appreciate digging into a lot of the conversations and concerns around this topic. I get a bit anxious when I don't understand something and the OCD side of me is triggered to dive through information and seek to uncover further information. Three points of discussion around higher red meat diets have surfaced over the past several decades that are fairly mainstream. I want to dive further in.

TMAO

In 2011 researchers published a paper linking the compound trimethylamine N-oxide (TMAO) to cardiovascular disease (CVD). Since then further research has confounded TMAOs role in pathology.

TMAO is a metabolite produced by gut microbes from dietary substrates (choline is a big one) found in animal foods. Once formed, it's transported to tissues where it can build up, while some is cleared by the kidneys.

There's several mechanisms by which researchers believe TMAO is linked to increased CVD, one of the main ones involves forming foam cells. The formation of these cells can disrupt cholesterol influx, esterification, efflux, and promote inflammation.

Initially this caused doctors to advise against the consumption of red meat, which can lead to more TMAO. Without going into lengthy detail, after reviewing the researchers methods there have been many flaws in the "links" theorized.'

For example, fish and other seafood contain the highest amounts of free TMAO, yet studies have found these foods actually **LOWER CVD**. Some have claimed the omega-3 fatty acids offset the impacts of TMAO. But we really don't have conclusive evidence to state one way or the other.

Conclusion, we just don't have conclusive evidence either way. And there's clear contradictory evidence.

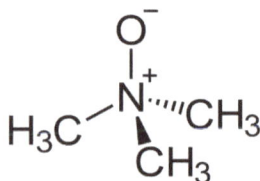

Image: TMAO molecule

mTOR

As you can see from the diagram above the mTOR mechanism is a bit complex to explain it in detail but essentially it is a protein enzyme that helps with cellular growth.

mTOR is necessary to build muscle. It is much more active in our early developmental stages as we're growing into human adults. We want it activated at times to allow our bodies to build up, but having it activate on all the time can lead to negative effects.

Studies have shown decreasing mTOR activation has been confirmed to increase lifespan in mice. It can slow the proliferation of cancer / rogue cells, and this makes sense since it's a complex necessary for cell growth, whether cancerous or healthy. Dietary regimens such as caloric restriction and methionine restriction can cause lifespan extension by decreasing mTOR activity.

So what's the big deal with mTOR in Carnivore?

Leucine vs Insulin

Meat is rich in leucine - an essential amino acid linked with a rapid stimulation and activation of mTOR. *Because of this and the above concerns around negative cell proliferation researchers and doctors have vilified the consumption of a high meat diet to minimize this. Interestingly though insulin stimulates mTOR for an even longer period of time.* Yet those same researchers do not trumpet restricting carbohydrates.

When we compare the meat triggering leucine to carbohydrate triggering insulin and how they impact mTOR, studies show the window of which mTOR is stimulated is higher when activated from insulin. [21]

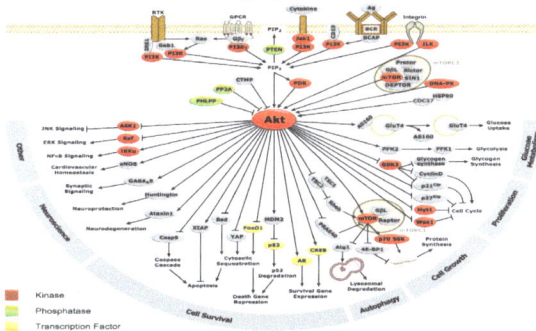

Image: mTor Complex Process

So if insulin is just as potent an mTOR activator and mTOR is activated longer than Leucine, why are we only vilifying meat?

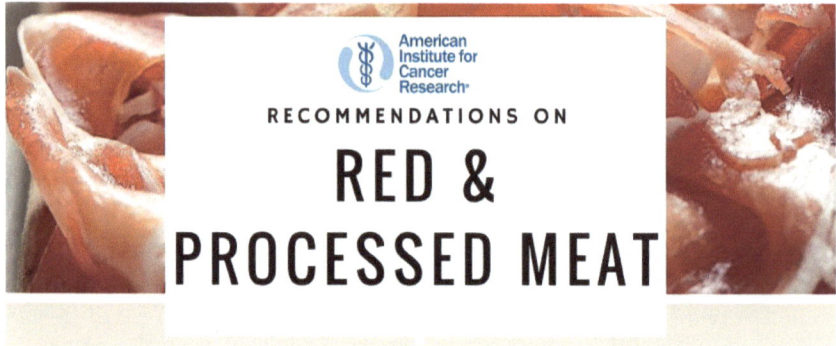

Cancer

This section could be an entire book in and of itself. I considered not even discussing it, but let's touch on it briefly. Keep in mind diving deep into the sciences and pursuing further reading and writing on this topic is beyond this scope of this text.

Over the last several decades "studies" have come out claiming red meat is carcinogenic. In particular individuals have pointed towards studies such as this [22] which are meta analyses (summaries) of a coll
ection of studies that are **epidemiological**. Formulating results and theories from epidemiology without interventional and control studies often leads to inaccurate and misleading information.

When you dive into the science and look for interventional or actual controlled research on the effects of red meat causing cancer, it becomes much less obvious that it is red meat causing it.

Grass fed beef is arguably one of the most nutritious foods a human being could possibly consume. [23] It contains CLA, electrolytes, complete protein, omega-3 fats, vitamin E content, lower levels of LDL (I'd argue elevated LDL may not even be a concern in the context of a metabolically healthy individual). 8 oz of grass fed beef contains: [59]

Amounts per 1 steak (214g)

Calorie Information

Amounts Per Selected Serving		%DV
Calories	250 (1047 kJ)	13%
From Carbohydrate	1.2 (5.0 kJ)	
From Fat	51.8 (217 kJ)	
From Protein	197 (825 kJ)	
From Alcohol	0.0 (0.0 kJ)	

Fats & Fatty Acids

Amounts Per Selected Serving		%DV
Total Fat	5.8 g	9%
Saturated Fat	2.2 g	11%
Monounsaturated Fat	2.1 g	
Polyunsaturated Fat	0.2 g	
Total trans fatty acids	0.2 g	
Total trans-monoenoic fatty acids	0.2 g	
Total trans-polyenoic fatty acids	0.0 g	
Total Omega-3 fatty acids	44.9 mg	
Total Omega-6 fatty acids	171 mg	

Protein & Amino Acids

Amounts Per Selected Serving		%DV
Protein	49.4 g	99%

Vitamins

Amounts Per Selected Serving		%DV
Vitamin A	0.0 IU	0%
Vitamin C	0.0 mg	0%
Vitamin D	~	~
Vitamin E (Alpha Tocopherol)	0.5 mg	2%
Vitamin K	1.9 mcg	2%
Thiamin	0.1 mg	7%
Riboflavin	0.3 mg	16%
Niacin	14.3 mg	72%
Vitamin B6	1.4 mg	70%
Folate	27.8 mcg	7%
Vitamin B12	2.7 mcg	45%
Pantothenic Acid	1.5 mg	15%
Choline	139 mg	
Betaine	16.3 mg	

Sterols

Amounts Per Selected Serving		%DV
Cholesterol	118 mg	39%
Phytosterols	~	

Carbohydrates

Amounts Per Selected Serving		%DV
Total Carbohydrate	0.0 g	0%
Dietary Fiber	0.0 g	0%
Starch	0.0 g	
Sugars	0.0 g	

Minerals

Amounts Per Selected Serving		%DV
Calcium	19.3 mg	2%
Iron	4.0 mg	22%
Magnesium	49.2 mg	12%
Phosphorus	454 mg	45%
Potassium	732 mg	21%
Sodium	118 mg	5%
Zinc	7.7 mg	52%
Copper	0.1 mg	7%
Manganese	0.0 mg	1%
Selenium	45.1 mcg	64%
Fluoride	~	

Other

Amounts Per Selected Serving		%DV
Alcohol	0.0 g	
Water	157 g	
Ash	3.6 g	
Caffeine	0.0 mg	
Theobromine	0.0 mg	

Image: Nutrition facts of grass fed steak

There's no question, this is a nutritional powerhouse for the human body. High quality grass fed beef comes with many additional nutrients we will discuss later in the book.

- 50 grams of protein (in the most bioavailable/digestible form)
- 45mg of omega-3 fatty acids
- 0.3 mg Riboflavin (16% DV)
- 14.3 mg Niacin (72% DV)
- 1.4mg Vitamin B6 (70% DV)
- 1.5mg Pantothenic Acid (15% DV)
- 139 mg Choline
- 4mg Heme Iron (22% DV)
- 49mg Magnesium (12% DV)
- 454mg Phosphorus (45% DV)
- 732mg Potassium (21% DV)
- 7.7mg Zinc (52% DV)
- 45 mcg Selenium (64% DV)

8OZ OF GRASS FED BEEF CONTAINS:

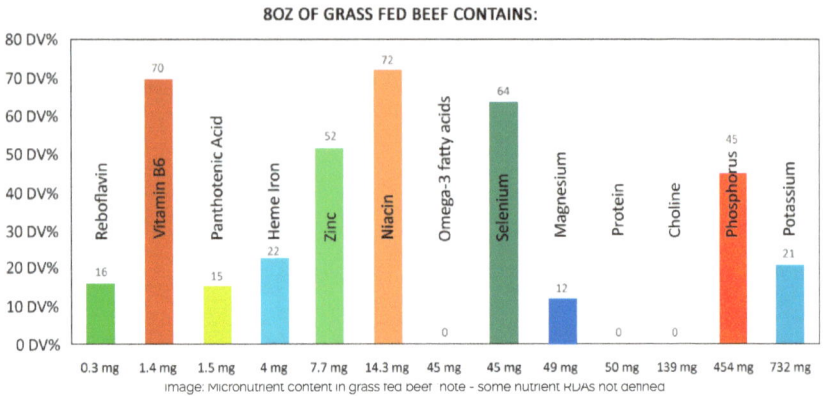

Reboflavin 16	Vitamin B6 70	Panthotenic Acid	Heme Iron 22	Zinc 52	Niacin 72	Omega-3 fatty acids 0	Selenium 64	Magnesium 12	Protein 0	Choline 0	Phosphorus 45	Potassium 21
0.3 mg	1.4 mg	1.5 mg	4 mg	7.7 mg	14.3 mg	45 mg	45 mg	49 mg	50 mg	139 mg	454 mg	732 mg

image: Micronutrient content in grass fed beef note - some nutrient RDAs not defined

Shaky research, at best, largely coming from epidemiology, along with nutritional profiles that are low in inflammation and autoimmune response and biochemically highly absorbable for humans makes classifying red meat as carcinogenic very hard to accept.

Another example of this is the case of sun exposure. One may decrease their risk for developing melona skin cancer by completely avoiding the sun. But we now know that there are tremendous health benefits and reductions in other much higher probable cancers that the UVB/UVA spectrums of light exposure from the sun help with avoiding.

The relatively weak scientific studies and the ample quality of nutrition through the unique and undeniable benefits of grass fed beef make it hard to accept it being carcinogenic. Its net effect is much more likely to prevent than cause cancer in humans who consume it.

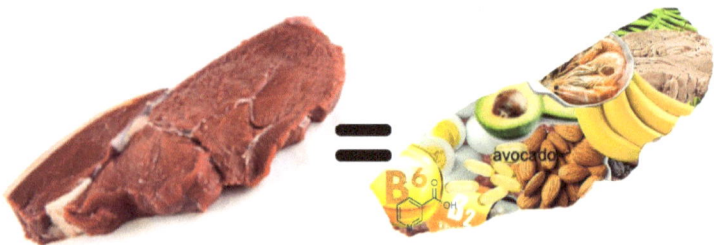

image: Steak and plant nutrient comparisons

8. LIPIDS, AND METABOLIC HEALTH

Cholesterol is a much more complex topic than researchers have made it out to be. When scientists started studying heart disease they noticed a correlation of higher cholesterol levels in patients who had hardened, clogged arteries, as well increased heart attacks, cardiovascular disease, and strokes.

Because elevated levels of cholesterol show up along with other markers present at the scene of these victims, they immediately vilified it. Cholesterol is often at the scene of the disease, but much less likely the cause.

Cholesterol is a waxy substance only produced by animals and humans. Plants do not have it. It's in every cell in the body and critical for cell membrane health.

When humans switch over to a fat-adapted ketogenic diet, their bodies are primarily running on ketone bodies from fat. Energy is transported to the cells through blood, but fat and blood are like oil and water. Fat doesn't mix well with blood and the body produces what are called lipoproteins to allow fat to be effectively transported.

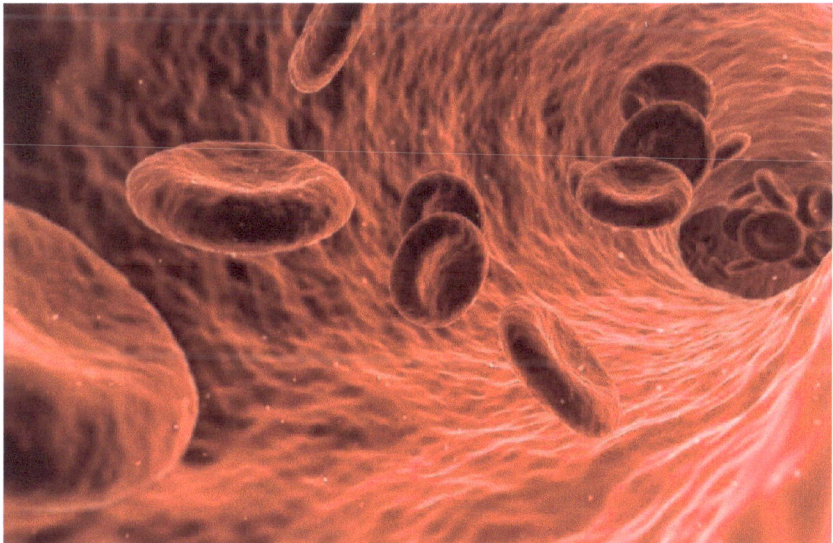

https://strokeprevention.info/risk-factor-high-cholesterol/cholesterol-is-stroke-in-your-blood/

Sadly, doctors and scientists still have very little understanding on this entire topic. We see people with totally clogged arteries who have perfectly normal functioning hearts. While high levels of cholesterol flow through both veins and arteries only plaque forms in the latter. How could this be, isn't cholesterol causing the plaque?

Constantin Velican, a notable researcher in the study of atherosclerosis with over 300 published, peer reviewed articles on heart disease stated, "no single etiological agent and pathogenetic mechanism have been clearly implicated as yet in the onset of early lesions in human coronary arteries. Also no useful result was reached during an entire century by continuing to put forward one theory [the cholesterol hypothesis] to the exclusion of others"

From my perspective I believe there are two main concerning factors you must watch with respect to lipids:

" I wouldn't be here if it weren't for a tremendous story that deeply impacted my life. This is the story of how I discovered the Carnivore Diet and how all of this came to be ".

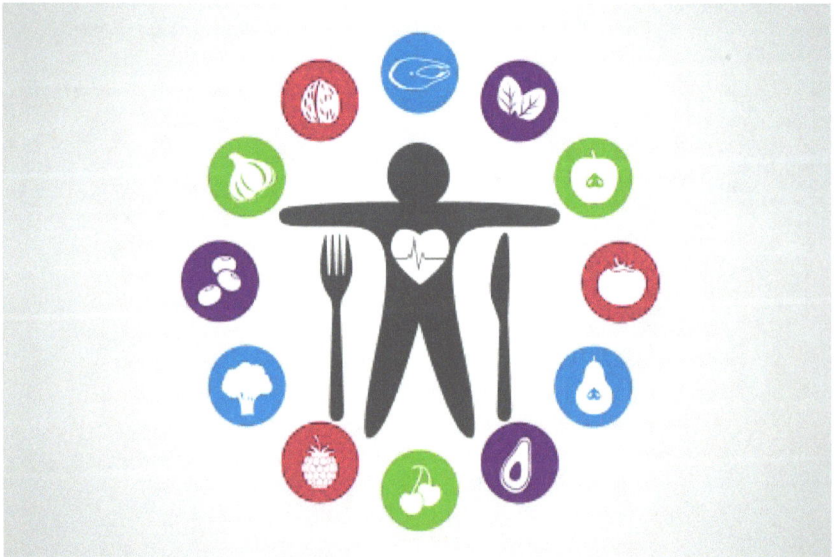

https://thebiostation.com/bioblog/fitness/5-ways-to-improve-your-metabolic-health/

1. Inflammation and Metabolic Dysfunction

What is most likely clear is if you have clear markers of metabolic dysfunction in the presence of elevated lipids - markers such as high fasted triglycerides, high inflammation (MPO and hs-CRP), elevated fasted insulin, high fasted glucose, even a high waist to height ratio (more subcutaneous visceral fat around your belly region), these are **much more indicative of disease and dysfunction** than purely looking at lipids alone.

When looking at heart health, doctors often want to see what's called a "lipid panel" to see the numbers of particles of lipoproteins to get a measure for total cholesterol. As mentioned above, lipoproteins are the molecules the body uses to move around the fat and cholesterol particles in the blood.

Test Name	Current Result & Relative Risk		Reference Range/Relative Risk Categories			
	Optimal	Non-Optimal	Optimal	Moderate	High	Units
METABOLIC						
Glucose[1]	79		65-99	100-125	<65 OR ≥126	mg/dL
Insulin	<1.0		≤19.6	N/A	>19.6	uIU/mL
HbA1c	5.3		<5.7	5.7-6.4	>6.4	%
Estimated Average Glucose	105		<117	117-137	>137	mg/dL
Triglycerides	61		<150	150-199	≥200	mg/dL
INFLAMMATION						
Myeloperoxidase[8]	179		<470	470-539	≥540	pmol/L
hs-CRP[6]	<0.3		<1.0	1.0-3.0	>3.0	mg/L

Image: My fasted inflammation & metabolic markers after a year carnivore from Nov 2019

2. The Lipid Particle Size

Another perspective which may have some merit, is looking at each type of lipid and better understanding how they function in the body; and watching out for the smallest potentially oxidized lipids. Doctors often focus on LDL and call it the "bad" cholesterol. But it may actually be the average size of our LDL.

Let's briefly discuss the different particles of cholesterol, what they do and then break down the concerns.

High Density Lipoproteins (HDL):

Produced by your liver and intestines contains more protein than fat, hence the name "high density." It has been touted as "good" cholesterol because it gathers up all cholesterol not being used by the body and returns it to the liver. Some studies have alluded that it helps with inflammation, immune regulation, diabetes and certain cancers. Having high HDL is generally considered good.

LIPIDS

Lipid Panel

Cholesterol, Total	303	<200	N/A	≥200	mg/dL
HDL Cholesterol	77	≥40	N/A	<40	mg/dL
Triglycerides	61	<150	150-199	≥200	mg/dL
LDL Cholesterol, Calculated	209	<100	100-129	>129	mg/dL (calc)
Chol/HDL-C	3.9	≤3.5	3.6-5.0	>5.0	calc
Non-HDL Cholesterol	226	<130	130-189	≥190	mg/dL (calc)
TG/HDL-C	0.8	<2.0	2.0-3.0	>3.0	calc
Lipoprotein Fractionation, NMR					
LDL-P[10]	2455	<935	935-1816	>1816	nmol/L
Small LDL-P	452	<467	467-820	>820	nmol/L
LDL Size	21.7	>20.5	N/A	≤20.5	nm
HDL-P	44.4	>32.8	29.2-32.8	<29.2	umol/L
Large HDL-P	14.9	>7.2	5.3-7.2	<5.3	umol/L

Test Name	Current		Reference Range/Relative Risk Categories			
	Result & Relative Risk		Optimal	Moderate	High	Units
	Optimal	Non-Optimal				
HDL Size	9.8		>9.0	8.7-9.0	<8.7	nm
Large VLDL-P	<1.5		<3.7	3.7-6.1	>6.1	nmol/L
VLDL Size	45.3		<47.1	47.1-49.0	>49.0	nm

Image: Kurt's blood nuclear magnetic resonance (NMR) lipid panel Nov 2019, 12 months Carnivore

Low Density Lipoproteins (LDL): LDL particles deliver nutrients and energy to cells. They move slower than HDL and can get stuck and oxidized. There "may", and this is a MASSIVE "may," be a link of these stuck particles contributing to plaque buildup in arteries. We think potentially the smaller LDL, not larger LDL particles, are more risky and want to know the average size.

Very Low Density Lipoproteins (VLDL): Even smaller potentially more likely to break - based on this hypothesis potential sticking and building up into the arteries.

Below I've shared my fasted lipid panel from November 2019, after a year of being on the Carnivore Diet. Notice my total cholesterol is "high" at 303 > 200 mg/dL, but HDL (good cholesterol) is 77 > 40. My fasted triglycerides are 61 > 150 is optimal. My LDL is 209 (bad cholesterol), but if you look at my particle sizes and VLDL, they all fall within the optimal sizes indicating, - if this theory is true, that I am in line with a lower risk profile and expected lipid profile for someone who is ketogenic.

This topic is becoming clearer, but we all still have much to learn. The good news is, for many, high lipids shouldn't be an alarm or solely indicate you are at risk.

For further deeper reading on this topic I recommend the following: Root Causing Health for their incredible work debunking myths of lipids and cardiovascular disease (CVD). Perfect keto and their blog headed by my friend Dr. Anthony Gustin. They do a great job breaking down more insight into how particle sizes may matter. Cholesterol Code is a helpful read on inflammation and cholesterol in general headed by engineer Dave Feldman for much deeper science on cholesterol.

— 9. THE VEGAN DILEMMA —
THE PLANET AND ANIMAL CRUELTY

It's not hard to see how attractive the vegan culture can be to the average consumer. It offers a "healthy" alternative that is better for animals, the planet and your overall vitality. Many people who shift from the standard american diet to a vegan diet feel an incredible "honeymoon phase" from the elimination of all the refined processed foods.

However, let's look into some of the biggest vegan claims and see if they actually measure up to their grandeur.

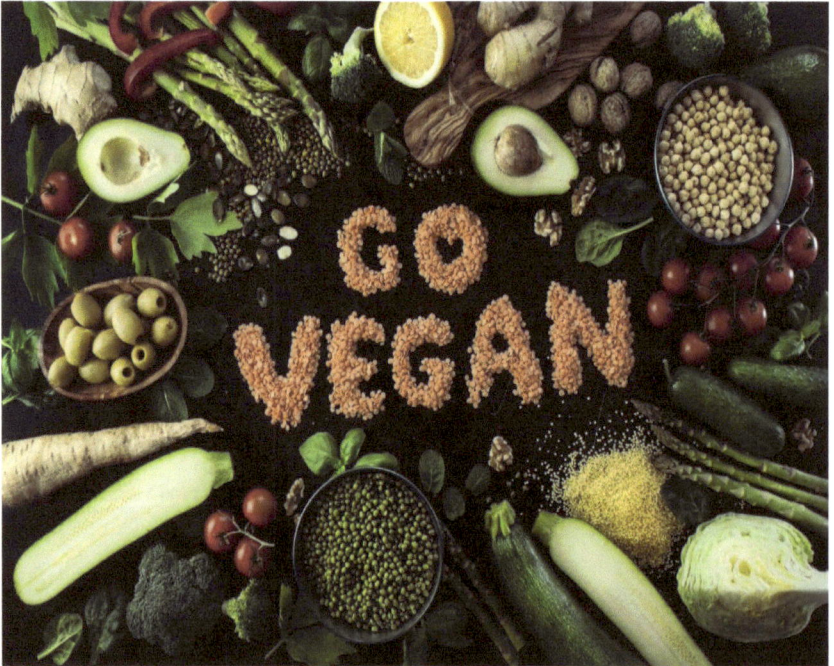

Image: Vegan vegetable images

Farming Methods

Factory farming, intensive methods designed to yield the maximum production while minimizing costs, is incredibly wasteful, destructive and cruel. We must all do our best to avoid purchasing and supporting these methods. If we look at all animal food as raised and created equal, without realizing that there is a nutritional difference and hefty impact on the environment and animals' lives (more to come later in the section on grass fed versus grain-fed,) we may indirectly be supporting these methods.

When looking at factory farming, it is quite easy to understand why many vegans are deeply opposed to animal foods. **These methods are cruel, wasteful and destroy natural ecosystems**. They are terrible and destructive.

We are all responsible for the health and future of this planet. I encourage everyone to learn more and to vote with their dollars by avoiding buying products from these mass operations utilizing these methods. In a world run by economics where monetary currency is exchanged for goods, factory farming fits very well for the average consumer.

We must recognize that these methods of agriculture, whether for animal or plant monocropping, cannot last and are not sustainable for the planet.

Many vegans take this to an extreme and translate a subset of factory farming practices across an entire industry. Their generalization is quite fair, but it is still a generalization and we have control to choose where our dollars go.

There are plenty of amazing farming practices where there exists incredible, regenerative, sustainable animal agriculture that is natural and healing to the planet.

Extreme vegan advocates will have many believe that plant foods are the only way to maintain a sustainable planet earth. They believe consuming animal foods is not only supporting animal cruelty, but also destroying the planet and human health. [24]

Overall Planet Greenhouse Gases

Let's look first at the planet. According to the EPA animal agriculture amounts to just 4% of carbon emissions. [25] Plant agriculture actually produces greater carbon emissions at 5%. Nearly 65% is from the burning of fossil fuels and industrial processes. Additionally the health care pharmaceutical industry is larger than that of livestock. [26]

Water & Land Use

Plant advocates argue animals take up an enormous amount of land and water usage. Many state that a single cow requires 280 gallons of water for every pound of produced meat. This land/water usage is less than the amount used for avocados, walnuts or sugar. But 94% (97% if grass finished) of water allocated to beef production **is naturally occuring rain water**. The overwhelming majority of the water would've fallen into the land regardless of whether or not cattle were there.

Land use is quite interesting. There are suggestions that ruminant animals such as livestock "waste" the land and produce a meager amount of calories for the space they consume.

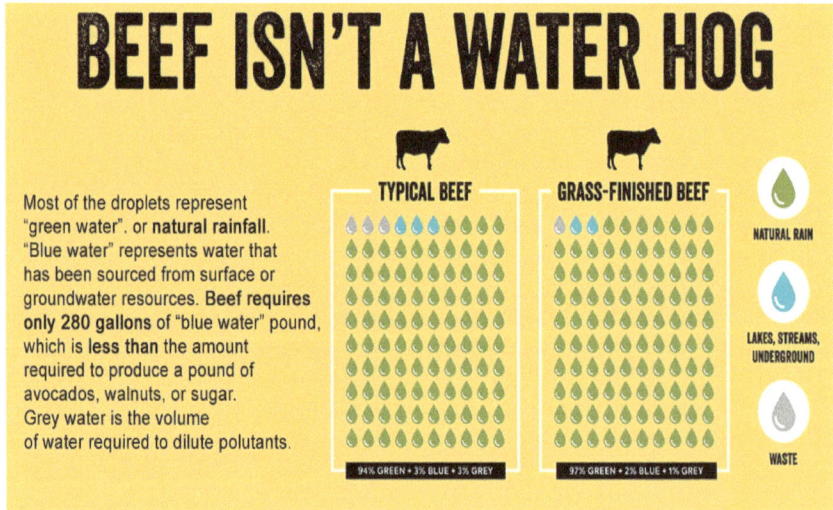

BEEF ISN'T A WATER HOG

TYPICAL BEEF   GRASS-FINISHED BEEF

Most of the droplets represent "green water", or **natural rainfall**. "Blue water" represents water that has been sourced from surface or groundwater resources. **Beef requires only 280 gallons** of "blue water" pound, which is **less than** the amount required to produce a pound of avocados, walnuts, or sugar. Grey water is the volume of water required to dilute polutants.

94% GREEN + 3% BLUE + 3% GREY   97% GREEN + 2% BLUE + 1% GREY

NATURAL RAIN

LAKES, STREAMS, UNDERGROUND

WASTE

Image Source: sacredcow.info

Holistic Management

I'd point you towards the works of Peter Ballerstedt [27] and Allan Savory [28], both of whom have spent decades and careers focusing on and understanding land and animal interaction. What we actually see is that herding animals are essential for soil health and replenishment. When the herds urinate, pass feces and compress that material into the land, it sequesters carbon, nutrients and allows for growable soil that would otherwise waste away.

I recently had the great pleasure of visiting White Oak Pastures [29], a farm practicing regenerative agriculture. They've done studies to show that their carbon footprint is net negative. They are actually improving the quality of the soil, the air and the environment.

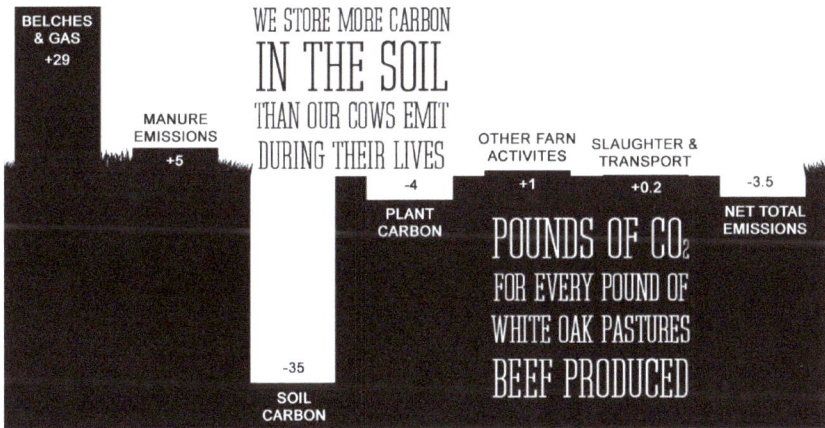

Image source: WhiteOakPastures.com

Animals evolved on our planet in an ecosystem over millions of years and replenish a cycle to graze the lands, sequester their waste. It's only when we change this process that we start to see problems.

Monocrop plant agriculture is arguably one of the most destructive of all types of farming methods. Whether we're stuffing livestock into massive feedlots or growing certain plant foods, we are not allowing the natural cycle of animals and their grazing on land to properly replenish the soil and nutrients. This depletes the soil, it's mineral content and the quality of the plant food grown on it.

Re-visiting the agricultural aspect, we have a substantial amount of plant-based agriculture accounting for much of this destruction. Soy and rice are the biggest proponents of these types of products.

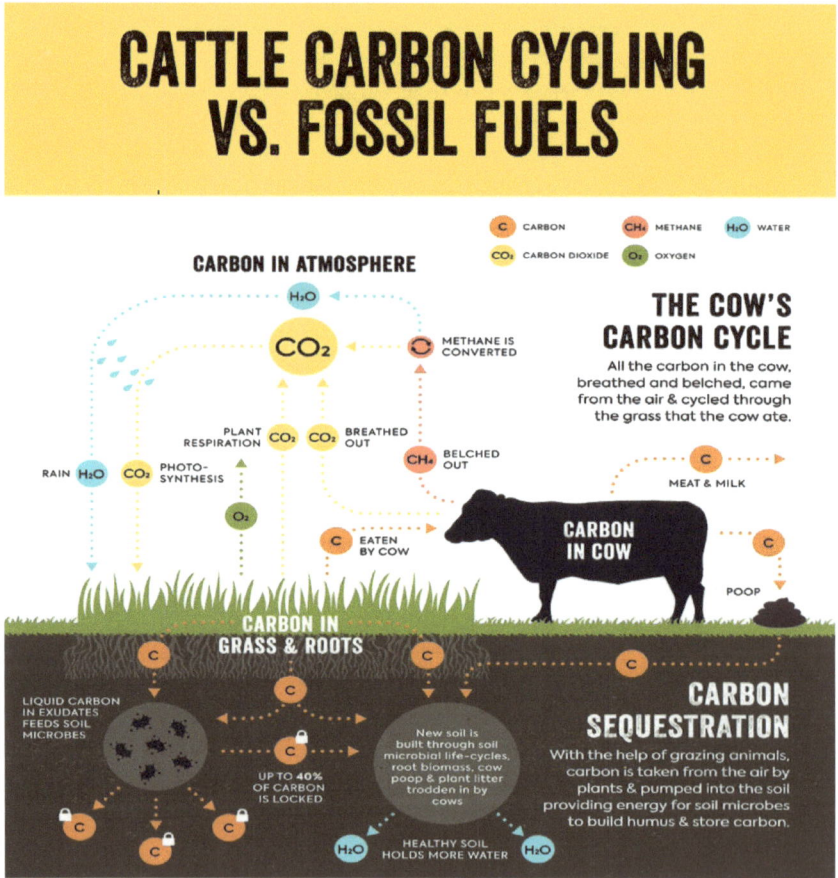

CATTLE CARBON CYCLING VS. FOSSIL FUELS

C CARBON   CH₄ METHANE   H₂O WATER
CO₂ CARBON DIOXIDE   O₂ OXYGEN

CARBON IN ATMOSPHERE

THE COW'S CARBON CYCLE

All the carbon in the cow, breathed and belched, came from the air & cycled through the grass that the cow ate.

H₂O

CO₂

METHANE IS CONVERTED

PLANT RESPIRATION CO₂   CO₂ BREATHED OUT

RAIN H₂O   CO₂   PHOTO-SYNTHESIS

CH₄ BELCHED OUT

MEAT & MILK

O₂

C EATEN BY COW

CARBON IN COW

C

POOP

CARBON IN GRASS & ROOTS

CARBON SEQUESTRATION

With the help of grazing animals, carbon is taken from the air by plants & pumped into the soil providing energy for soil microbes to build humus & store carbon.

LIQUID CARBON IN EXUDATES FEEDS SOIL MICROBES

New soil is built through soil microbial life-cycles, root biomass, cow poop & plant litter trodden in by cows

UP TO 40% OF CARBON IS LOCKED

H₂O HEALTHY SOIL HOLDS MORE WATER H₂O

Image Source: sacredcow.info

The answer is not to eliminate consumption of nutrient-rich animals that graze these lands, but rather to create and support the natural lifecycle and sustainability of the process that has been in existence for millennia before modern farming practices came into the picture.

The Cost of Going "Green"

I'll add that a LARGE proportion of a plant-based diet often comes from foods not native to the consumer. Virtually all fruit consumed is shipped over 1,000's of miles to reach you. A banana for breakfast likely comes from Ecuador or somewhere else in South America. The only state in the US that grows coffee is Hawaii. Yet we drink it knowing it's shipped across hundreds, if not thousands of miles. **The carbon footprint of the many diverse plants is not small**. Avocados and almonds are massive consumers of non-natural water. The soy industry [30] is one of the largest factors of deforestation in South America.

Animal Cruelty

Another reason many are abstaining from animal products is to limit animal suffering. Sadly, this is far from the case - *there is a titanic volume of death that accompanies traditional plant-farming methods. The soil tilling destroys most of what naturally exists prior to planting. Pesticides are sprayed across large acres of crops to kill off the insects and animals that feed on these crops.* In addition, rodents and predators lured in to these massive traps of "food" are shot on sight.

To say that plant agriculture eliminates death and suffering is a false narrative. I'm not saying one side is at fault here. But claiming you're ending animal suffering by eating plant foods, and not eating animals that were killed to grow those crops, is naive or hypocritical. The reality is the planet needs both animals and plants to sustain the carbon cycle and maintain healthy soil. Life and death are a natural process of nature. We humans too will be consumed by plants, and then animals one day.

Humans greatly benefit from the nutrition of wholesome animal foods. As a society we need to become aware of where, and how, our food is coming to us and take up efforts to support the farmers and providers who really care about these factors.

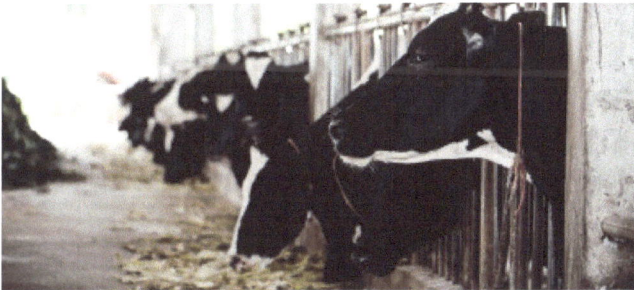

Image Source: freepik.com

10. PREGNANCY
AND BREASTFEEDING

Disclaimer 1

I wish I could take full responsibility to tell you to listen to me. Personally I would absolutely follow this advice with my own child and family but I have to say **I'm not a doctor**. Always check your doctor prior to pursuing any sort of changes to your diet and health regimen or when following a unique diet, especially during pregnancy.

Disclaimer 2

If you're not already on a ketogenic and/ or Carnivore Diet, pregnancy is NOT the time to try to do one. Changing your diet can stress your body. It can change your hormones and affect a lot of variables as it adjusts. Unless you're dealing with serious complications and your doctor is advising you to do so, learn and practice this way of eating before you get pregnant.

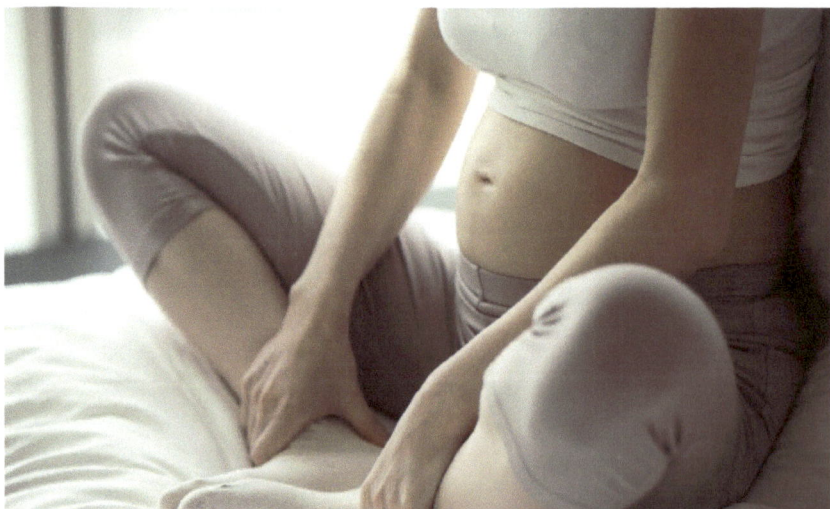

Image Source: freepik.com

Now nto the meat of this section! Is the Carnivore Diet really safe and what and how do we know? Well, after digging around the web looking through studies and articles, I found there are very few trials done on ketogenic diets and pregnancy.

" I wouldn't be here if it weren't for a tremendous story that deeply impacted my life. This is the story of how I discovered the Carnivore Diet and how all of this came to be ".

Study of Mice

There is only one study of pregnant mice. In that study mice were fed a "synthetic" ketogenic diet of Canola oil and crisco. No one would ever recommend giving that to a pregnant woman.

What they found was that the development of some of the fetus organs differed. The brain in particular was quite a bit larger. While others, such as the liver, were below size for the control group. The scientific abstract is here for reference. [48] From this study researchers concluded organs did not form properly and that a ketogenic diet may not be safe due to "abnormal" development of organs, which could cause complications later in child / adult development.

Image: Ketosis vs Ketoacidosis

Dietary Ketosis vs Ketoacidosis

Another reason for doctors to be concerned is that they may be mixing up dietary ketosis with diabetic ketoacidosis. Humans run on ketones when starved. One is a metabolically healthy state taking in sufficient calories while the other is a dangerous state where blood ketones build up creating an overly high acidic state within the blood. This happens almost exclusively to type 1, and less commonly type 2 diabetics. Rarely is there ever a case for a metabolically healthy woman.

When doctors hear this term they can be trained and thinking you're starving yourself, or become concerned for elevated acid levels in the blood. Instead of seeing a **well-formulated low carb diet**, they consider a pregnant woman who is starved, and this creates valid concerns. That said, consuming a diet rich in wholesome foods and rich in healthy natural fats, with well-balanced vitamins, is ideal for a pregnant woman.

Treating PCOS with Keto Diets

The third point I want to bring up is that we see improved fertility with high fat diets for women. Studies show fertility improves, Polycystic Ovary Syndrome (PCOS), which impacts ovulation, can have a strong impact on one's ability to get pregnant. It's largely believed to exist from the experience of imbalanced hormones, elevated male hormones in particular. In a study conducted in 6 groups, 5 groups reported improved fertility on a low carb diet. The study also concluded that lowering carbs could impact lowering insulin levels, help balance hormones and improve pregnancy rates compared to a regular diet. When women go on a low carb diet, often elevated insulin levels, triglycerides and hormones are given a chance to return to normal ranges.

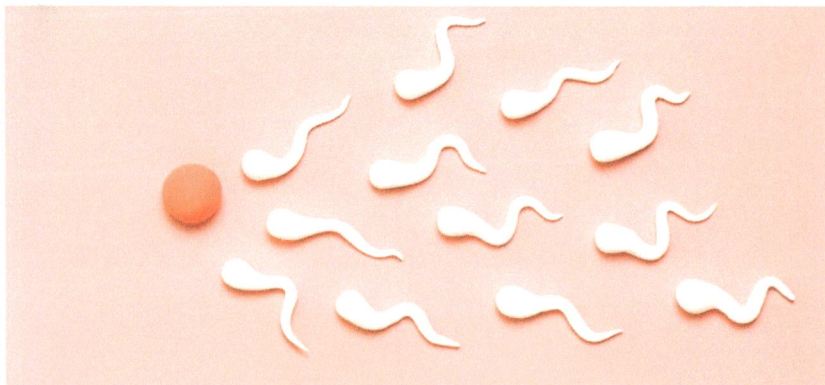

Image: Ketosis vs Ketoacidosis

Healthy Fats Fuel Hormones

A ketogenic whole food diet contains a lot of fats. The Carnivore Diet diet provides the body with key building blocks it needed to create hormones. The brain of the baby is the fattiest organ, largely composed of fat and cholesterol.

Ancestral and Biological Alignment

Why would nature make the body **more fertile, in some cases fix infertility, if the cause** of what's actually doing that, **were harmful to a baby?** It just doesn't seem to make a lot of sense. Early in pregnancy women become more insulin resistant. This increases their appetite hyperplasia and increased lipogenesis (the breakdown of fat). It appears their body wants increased calories and fats rich in fat-soluble vitamins which are an excellent source of nutrients for the baby's large head - which is full of brains. Brains are made up of cholesterol, fat and some protein. Ancestrally pregnant women would eat the fat and micronutrient rich organs such as liver and kidney.

Breastfeeding:

Infants are born in a natural state of ketosis. They maintain this healthy state while breastfeeding. A mother's breast milk is ~ 50-60% fat and almost 6x the dietary cholesterol adults typically get. It's also loaded with Ancel Keys's notoriously dangerous saturated fat.

Understandably we haven't conducted studies with pregnant women in this area. Ketogenic diets can leave women under-eating due to the level of satiety of the nutrient dense foods. So they must work closely with their doctor and make sure they are getting sufficient calories. Pregnancy is not the time to go into a caloric deficit.

Under-eating can lead to lack of calories and inadequate milk production. That said, as long as they're eating healthy wholesome foods and getting enough calories, there's quite a bit of anecdotal feedback showing that a high fat low carb diet is actually more beneficial in supporting healthy milk production. One study [60] found that a low carb, high fat diet, provided more energy in the milk for the baby. Daily calories required to produce a healthy breast milk supply - alone could be as much as 500-600 calories above your maintenance calorie range.

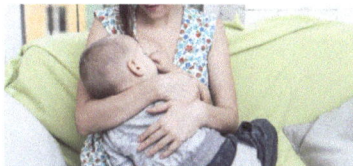

Image: freepik.com

11. EMOTIONS
OF EATING

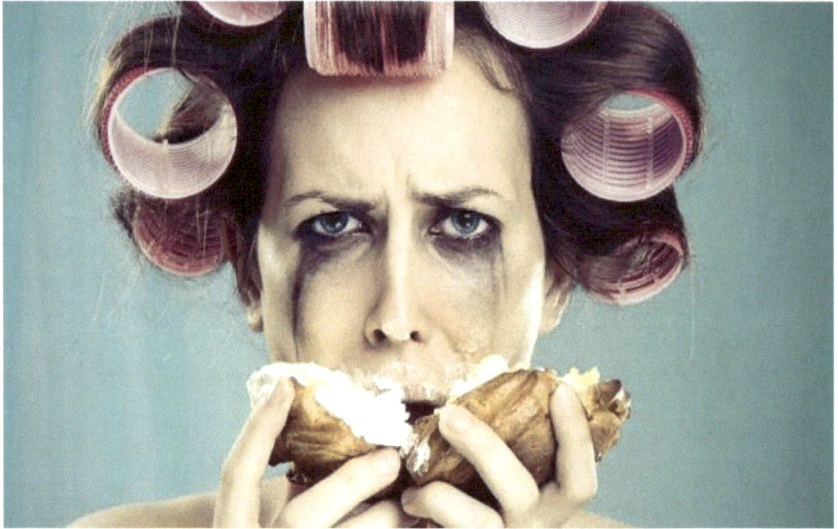

Image: Eating Emotionally

Three Brain Model (Triune), Psychology

The Carnivore Diet can seem extreme and overwhelming when first starting. Eliminating all fruits, veggies and spices, and restricting what you put in your body to meat and salt, is a drastic change for most.

Establish Your Why

Doing anything of great effort requires a great reason, a powerful why. Without a purpose, a clear reason for succeeding, you will struggle and there will be many reasons and opportunities to fall back to old habits and eating patterns. For me, coming from a place of chronic anxiety, depression and trauma was a constant pain and great motivator to find a way to feel better. I was driven by a powerful avoidance of significant discomfort and pain.

What is Your Story?

Human beings are extraordinarily adaptive. We can transform and make incredible changes. BUT we can only do so if we have reasons and significant motivation. Many of our previous life adaptations were forced through life or death situations. But now we have a comfortable world with incredible healthcare. We can mask symptoms and prop up our health through pharmaceutical interventions and medical treatments.

In order to conquer habits and human nature which have evolved over millions of years, it benefits us to look at some unique models and better understand how our brains, emotions and habits work

Triune Brain Model

This is a model of the brain that suggests there are actually three (tri) brains in a human being [31]. There is the Neocortex - rational thinking brain, the Limbic Brain - emotional feeling brain - and the Reptilian brain - instinctual dinosaur brain.

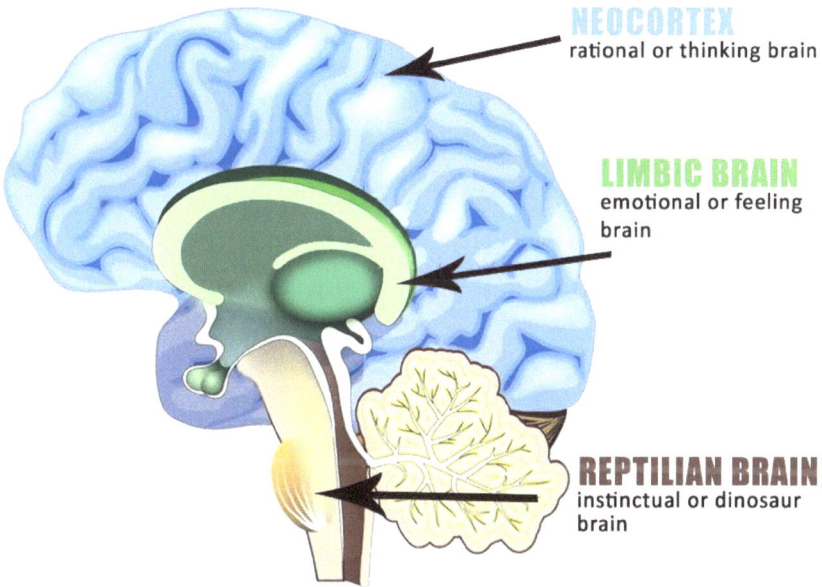

NEOCORTEX
rational or thinking brain

LIMBIC BRAIN
emotional or feeling brain

REPTILIAN BRAIN
instinctual or dinosaur brain

Image: Human brain and the three brains we evolved

Dr. McClean modeled that human beings need the lower, more primitive brain, and can not function and survive without the less advanced. The more primitive we go within the brain, the more essential to survival. When humans experience stress or trauma, our direction to function reverts to these lower more ancestral cores of thinking.

Our reptilian biology has us wired to seek out things that keep us safe and comfortable. Avoid death, eat, have sex and sleep. This is basically what your biology has been intelligently designed to do. These are instincts, not emotions.

As we became mammals and developed our limbic Brain, we learned to interact and "feel" emotions - a chemistry of familiar sensations we could label. Think for a moment about what anxiety is. Where do you feel it, at what intensity and in what way? Now think about excitement. How is excitement felt and experienced as sensations in your body? *Mammals became more intelligent by connecting themselves socially through their emotions.* A herd of several mammals could better collectively sense dangers and lead each other safely through operating and communicating with emotions as a collective.

In our more advanced stages of evolution we were given our "human" neocortex brain which could add in logic. It could comprehend, reason, and deduct information.

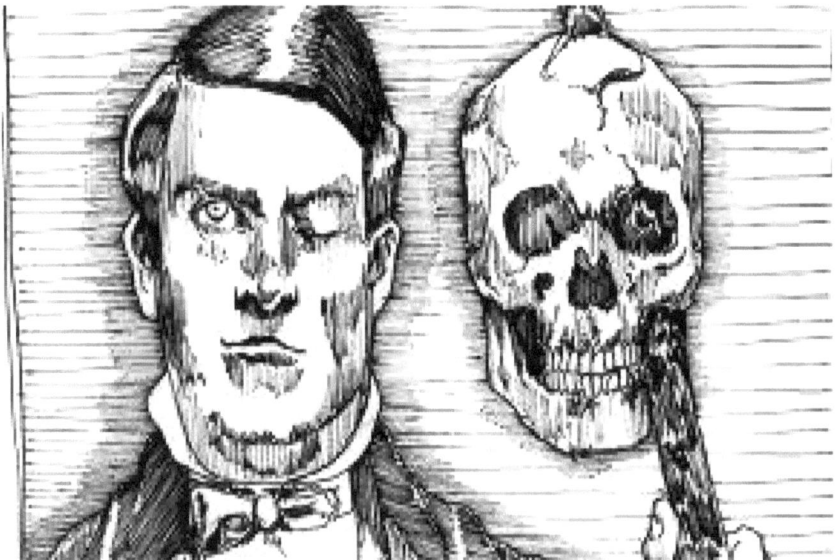

Image: Phineas Gage famous brain injury

Phineas Gage, railway worker who suffered traumatic brain injury, losing much of his left cerebrum but surviving and functioning more than a decade after.

Humans can survive without sections of the neocortex (human brain) or, limbic (mammalian brain). But damage to the reptilian brain results in severe physical disabilities and often death. We don't function optimally. Historical cases show that individuals experiencing brain injuries, depending on which part is removed typically experience a correlated impairment.

I explain all this to put into perspective that we are driven by deeper, more primal systems that must be respected. We are not simply beings with conscious, rational thoughts from which we can easily and quickly change. Learning and understanding this will help intelligently approach changing and rewiring the habits we've had for so long.

It also may be cause to explore deeper lying issues (in our mammalian brain) around safety and security that may be tied to emotional eating. [49] *The deeper driving forces that contribute to emotional eating are not logically or rationally driven.* They are driven by the systems and mechanisms that evolved over millions of years. They are deeper and more rooted in safety, survival and security.

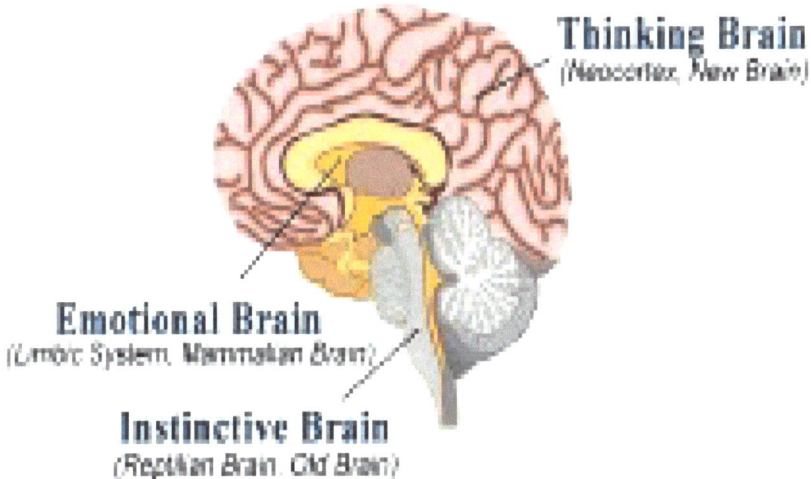

Thinking Brain
(Neocortex, New Brain)

Emotional Brain
(Limbic System, Mammalian Brain)

Instinctive Brain
(Reptilian Brain, Old Brain)

Image: https://www.southernmarylandchronicle.com/2019/02/18/mammalian-brain-like-youve-never-seen-it-before/

Emotional Mammalian Eating

When I was 24 I started studying hypnotherapy. I was turned on to it by a mentor while I was looking to make some major personal behavioral changes. One of the certification courses covered treatment protocols on emotional eating. The instructor explained a scenario which helped us better understand what was going on.

If someone experiences an abusive relationship with their partner, physical or emotional, one can often develop an eating disorder or indulge in habits to reduce their attractiveness so that their partner leaves them. Indirectly this makes them safer from that danger. The mind doesn't realize these habits may be causing long term health damage. It simply realizes that this action feels good and brings safety.

I share all this to put things in context. The human mind can be elusive and complex. It is built on archaic systems of brains that do not talk well to each other, with the purpose of protecting us at all costs. Understanding how these older,

more primal systems work, can help us see blind spots and reasons why we engage in destructive behaviors.

Awareness is a powerful skill. It can be extremely difficult to see our own blind spots, especially when we realize they're created by much older systems that evolved over millions of years to keep us alive, and avoid immediate threats.

Professional Help

If you believe you might be dealing with a deeper underlying issue that is causing you to eat in unhealthy ways, consider seeking professional help or counseling. There's no shame in admitting you have weaknesses and blindspots. Our egos often block us from becoming our best selves. Remember, the best performers in the world all have coaches. I can personally testify that I wouldn't be the person I am today if I hadn't invested in 1,000s of hours and $1,000s of dollars into personal therapy and coaching. The earlier I made those investments and the more investments I made, the more successful I have become.

So, if you feel you have strong reasons for change, and you feel solid about your emotions, understanding and ability to set goals to change habits, let's jump into it!

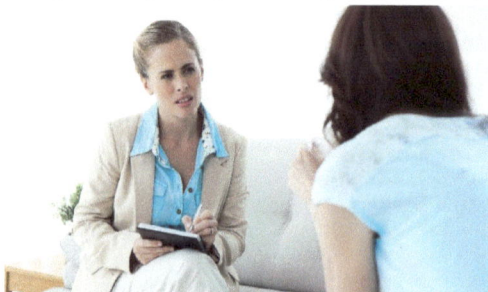

Image: Mental health professional counseling client

12. MINDSET
AND PROGRESSION

Starting the Carnivore Diet is simple, but probably not easy.

You'll be eliminating all plant molecules from your diet. That means no more spices and seasonings. You'll be focused on more nutrient dense, wholesome foods.

Don't worry! I've built out a detailed plan and approach to get us where we want to go. First I'll help you better understand more triggering and "tolerable" foods. Then we'll talk about the progression, and finally I'll provide simple, easy to make, low cost meal plans you can implement. For those of you who feel emotionally fit and ready. Let's dive in!

Mindset

Always remember WHY you're doing this. You MUST find a BIGGER reason than the pleasure of food to deeply connect with it. There will be days, **especially early on**, when you find yourself in a less than optimal emotional state. Those moments will test your will.

find your why
p u r p o s e   i s   k e y

Why

Below are some "why's" I've used to keep myself motivated and on the Carnivore Diet. I provide these as examples. You're welcome to use them or come up with your own. Just have one or two really solid "whys" you can reference and keep top of mind. The going early on can be a challenge and you'll want to be able to easily remind yourself of your reasons on those especially testing days:

1. My health is the single highest leverage driver I can improve to support accomplishing my dreams. When I'm healthy my focus is better, my energy and my ability to perform for myself and my team is greatly improved. When I snack and consume foods that negatively impact my mood, sleep and vitality, I see a direct negative impact on my performance and production.

2. I need to do this before disease tells me I MUST. I do not want to let disease be the message that forces me to change. I seek to improve the quality of my life and experience every day with more vitality and a higher mood through long term consumption of high quality food.

3. Carb-rich, sugary foods are addictive. I don't indulge in addictions and I don't enjoy short-term pleasures that negatively impact long term prosperity. Instead I prefer to work through long term dietary rewards.

4. I no longer eat for pleasure. I eat to fuel my body and long-term health. If these parts of me are compromised I am unable to truly support my mission of my biggest dreams.

5. The feeling I get from stable, steady, guilt-free nutrients entering my body and fueling my mood are enormous. When I stick to this, my vitality and the levels of energy I develop are tremendous.

6. I'll be a better parent, lover, leader, example to my child, spouse and teammate that will ultimately inspire others to live their best, most healthy lives.

7. My mother / father passed away from X. If I continue down the same pattern of lifestyle and diet I am putting myself at risk for much of the same.

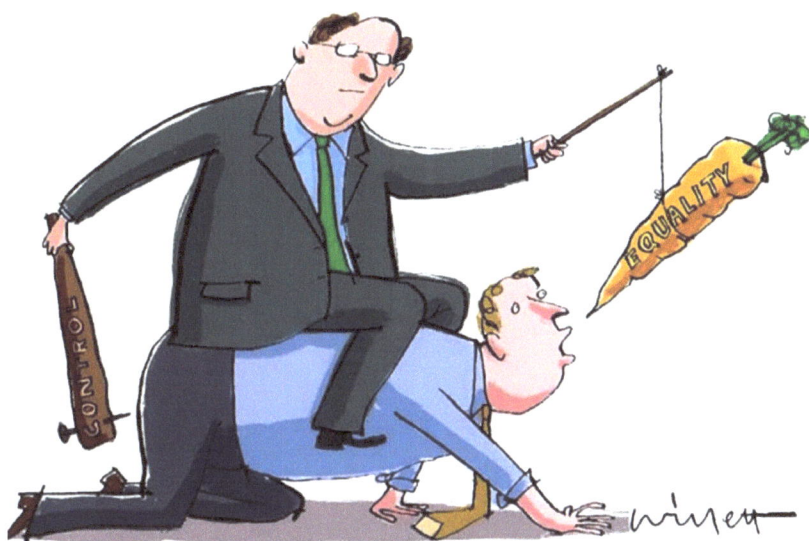

Image: the stick vs carrot incentives

The Stick

Ask yourself what you truly value in life. What has the most meaning in your life? Is it really the short-term pleasures of indulging in foods that damage your health and limit your human capacity? Remind yourself of all the pain that comes after you indulge. The guilt, the loss of self-respect, the reinforcement of a physique you do not desire.

The Carrot

Think about how great you'll feel when you can breathe clearly. Think about sleeping optimally. Think about not being on edge because you ate something that just isn't sitting well. Imagine no longer experiencing anxiety - even at a subtle level. How about having blood sugar and energy levels that are optimized and consistent?

The Trial

Remember you're not writing off "cheat" foods forever, you're just saying goodbye for a period of time. Maybe someday you'll come back. For now you're saying, "see you later" so you can see how healthy you can become. Remember how self-destructive off plan food can be and how you feel after eating that garbage.

Imagine what it would feel like if none of that was an issue, if none of your focus and energy were diverted that way. Imagine going through a day where you no longer worry about food. Think about that and instead, focus on moving towards your dreams, your goals, your mission and becoming a better leader for others that look up to you. What if you woke up feeling amazing, energized, vital, free of health issues and you could dive right into what is most meaningful to you? How could you feel about making serious progress towards attaining it?

What is the Compound Effect?

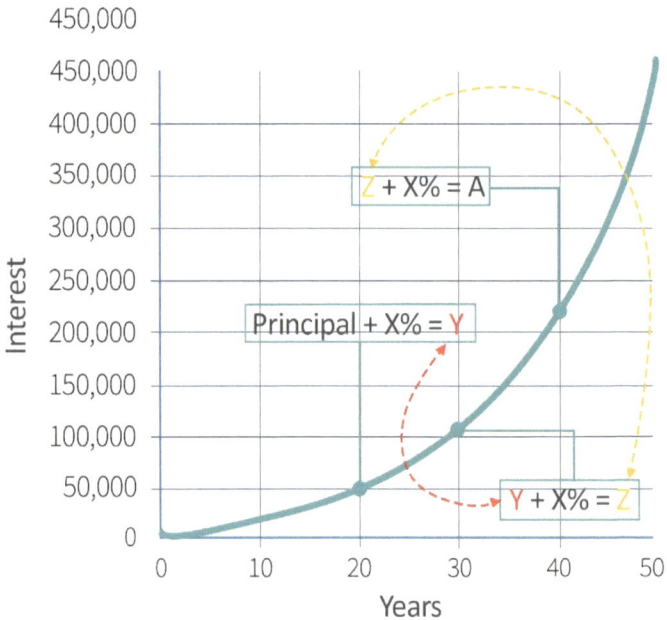

Z + X% = A

Principal + X% = Y

Y + X% = Z

Interest / Years

Image: Mental health professional counseling client

The Compound Effect

Einstein famously stated *compound interest is the most powerful force in the universe. "He who understands it, earns it, he who doesn't, pays it."*

Think about the detrimental compound effect of a brief indulgence (30 mins of flavor sensations), spiking dopamine (pleasure reward centers in your brain,) of eating less than optimal food, and the negative impact that can have on your ability to experience and be your best. Often the effect of a meal like this is so destructive to our cognitive and physical selves, we lose hours, days and in some cases, weeks of lost productivity and vitality. I'd argue the worst part is that our subjective judgement is impaired. We tell ourselves it really isn't that big of an impact. But in fact it can truly impair our cognitive and physical abilities.

Compound that with the time you spend in the aftermath and it's easy to see how much leverage one can gain or lose depending on mental states and abilities.

For many Carnivores it can take months to reverse the damage their diet has been causing them. I'm not saying this to discourage you from starting. Often there are exceptional benefits just days in. Many do see chronic symptoms substantially diminish or disappear very early on. But I do want to bring this to your awareness because the consequences of indulging can be quite devastating and they often have a compounding effect on your entire life.

When you bring to your awareness the full weight and full extent of destruction to which you are partaking, and you put that into perspective with what it is you truly value (health, vitality, steady energy, optimal cognition, being the best version of yourself), it becomes very clear where the priorities are. Life is very short. You're only here for a brief time.

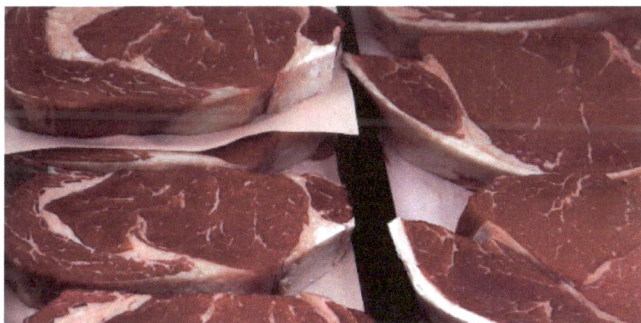

Image: https://foreignpolicy.com/2013/07/09/the-french-flicks-and-american-beef-standing-in-the-way-of-a-u-s-eu-trade-deal/

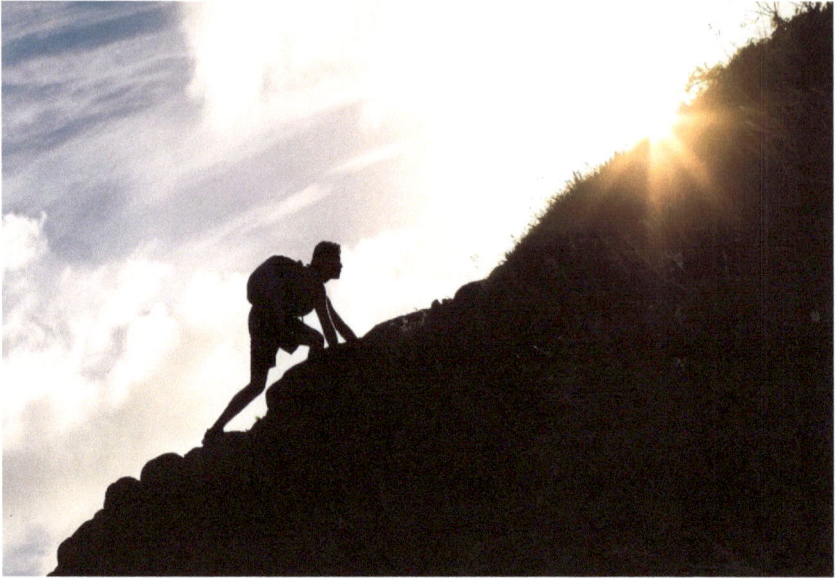

Image: Progressing up a climb

Progression

Keep in mind you don't have to do this diet all at once. *In fact, when I started I was still eating plant foods for several weeks before I totally weaned myself off my go-to snacks.* There are no good grades here for individuals who transition faster than others. Instead focus on how well you are with being consistent and stick to it long term.

Many people can eat a meat-heavy meal once in a while. But can you avoid that cake sitting on the counter someone brought in for the office? Are you able to skip ordering at the drive-thru when you're with your friends and they want to pick up some terrible fried food. (Remind yourself the price you pay for consuming that!)

These temptations are real. You're overcoming deep parts of your biology; emotional and instinctual systems hard-wired into your body over millions of years, designed to seek out short-term pleasures regardless of their long term benefits. *Be kind to yourself and realize that positive self-talk and reinforcement is the best way to make this transition.*

A. Eat more animal foods

Start with adding more animal foods. Take advantage of your nature to want to consume more and eat larger portions of animal foods. Add an extra egg, order that larger sized steak, burger or filet.

Prioritize animal foods. Eat all the animal foods on your plate first before finishing the veggies and fruits. Cut back on those spices and sauces that aren't fully animal based and often loaded with sugar.

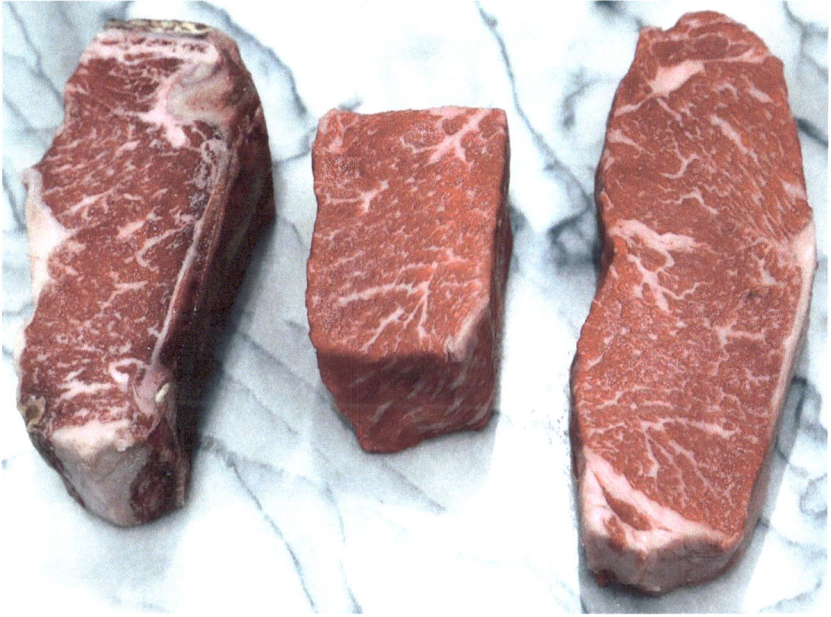

Image: Cuts of fatty beef

B. Think Low Carb

When you plan meals, start removing items that are starchier and higher in sugars and carbs. Leave out soda and juices, maybe not every day, but every few days, then every other day.

C. Stop Buying Those Cheats

A big part of new habit formation is creating resistance to indulge in existing habits. As you transition and finish off (or better yet, toss out) those cheat foods, consider NOT buying them next time you're at the grocery / market. If you don't have these items within reach - when you feel the urge - you'll have much more resistance to consume them freely because you'll have to go out and buy them.

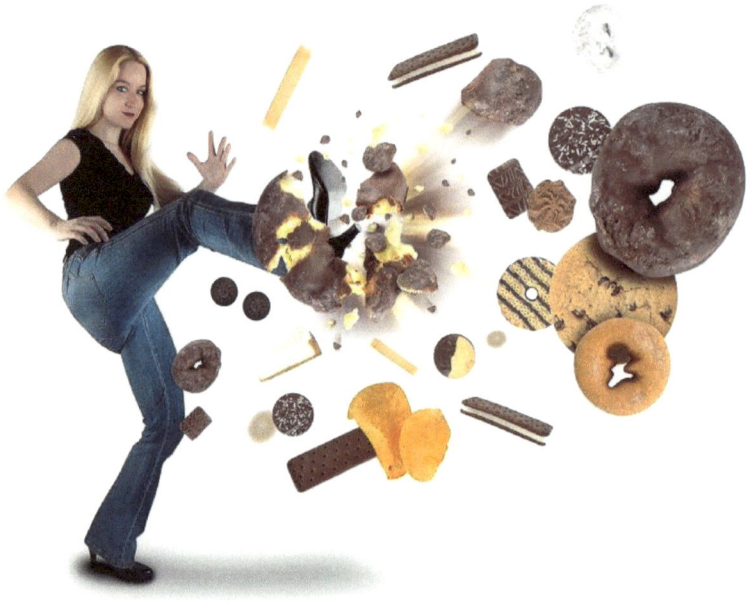

Image: Kicking bad foods and habits

D. Start planning food

Think about what you'll be eating a day or two prior. We humans aren't always in our peak emotional state. Often during the work week, during a particularly tough day, where we find ourselves tired and spent, we can reach for the easiest hunger and emotional relief. If you're having a particularly tough day you're going to reach for what's easy and emotionally "good" feeling. But if you plan and have carnivore items you can access, you'll be much more inclined to indulge in healthy eating.

Your plan doesn't have to be fancy and heavily thought out. Start with keeping a dozen eggs, some cut up meats and fat trimmings in the office fridge. These items along with a good knife, a cutting board and scale (all of which can be easily ordered online for reasonable costs), will equip you with more than enough for a solid Carnivore meal.

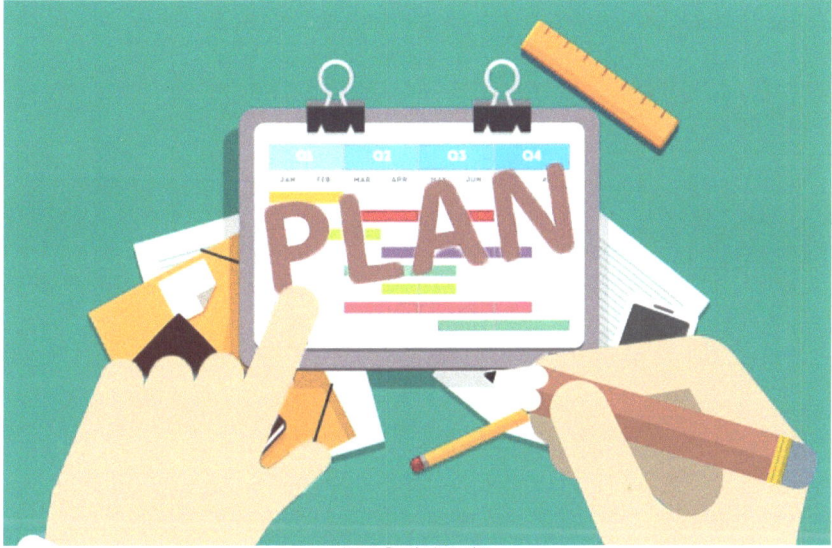

Image: Developing a plan

13. ADAPTATION
AND MEAL PLANNING

Most people will experience some symptoms of transition. These typically subside within a few days, to a few weeks, depending on the adaptation timeline, your physical condition and how your body responds.

Keto-flu symptoms such as headache, foggy brain, fatigue, irritability, nausea, difficulty sleeping and constipation are all common. [17] With respect to your gut and digestion - loose stool, diarrhea, weakness, fatigue, dry mouth, stress, bloating and some cramping may occur.

Hang in there though, this **DOES NOT** mean this diet is bad for you or that you're not doing it properly. Much of these symptoms are due to the change in our body's ability to process and absorb different energy and nutrients. Your body needs time to adjust. Bacteria between the small and large intestines need time to grow and shift to build up.

Mental

The gut and mind are tightly connected. The gut issues below are likely part of the mental symptoms you'll experience. Remember you are also removing the majority of carbohydrates (muscle meats do contain some carbs) from your diet. This drastic reduction requires adaptation. The body needs to shift and get used to lower levels of insulin and using ketones as fuel.

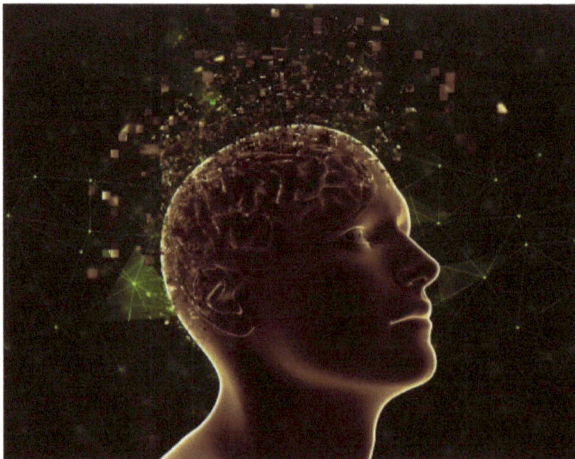

Image: freepik.com

Gut & Physical

You'll be introducing a much larger quantity of animal foods. This will be an adjustment to digestion as your small intestine is where you absorb the majority of these types of foods. Early on, with this new food type coming in, they will need to grow to meet the demands of the added volume of animal foods entering your small intestine. There will be a transition during this shift to build up "carnivore" bacteria to help breakdown and absorb these foods

The large intestine, colon and rectum are the last location food travels until expelled as waste. This is where the most difficult, fibrous foods (often plants) and any other food not taken up by the stomach and small intestine often get fermented with one last attempt at absorption. With the reduction and elimination of food typically entering this region, the bacteria in these parts of the digestive system will be starved.

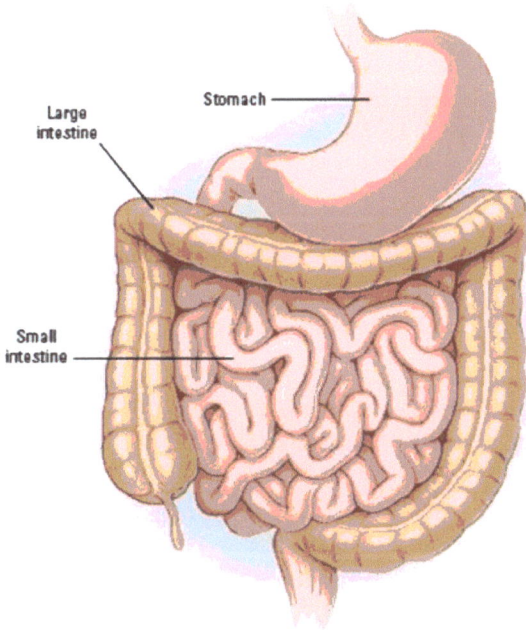

Image: Human gut, stomach, small and large intestinal tract

Loose Stool

When animal foods hit different regions of your gut without being fully absorbed, water can flow into those sections. Since a Carnivore Diet early on is likely front loading your stomach and small intestine with more volume than it's used to, food that normally wouldn't make it all the way to the large intestine often does. Combining that with water will often create diarrhea-like symptoms. Once the small intestine has adjusted and bacteria has built up to assist in breaking down those foods you'll see these symptoms subside.

Quick note - For some people, supplementing Betaine HCL (250-1,000mg) may help support their gut as they transition and/or during being Carnivore. With the increased amount of protein and fat entering the stomach this can help support the need for increased acid volume and concentration. Also consider avoiding excessive fluid consumption 20 mins prior to or after digestion.

Meal Plan

Let's discuss direct, actionable meal plans. In my personal experience there's really two approaches to take to do the diet. (a) [Gradual] Gradually shift over to a full Carnivore Diet over several weeks or (b) [Full On] Fully jump in to the diet right away.

The gradual shift will likely make more sense for individuals who:

A. Are skeptical and lack confidence in following a strict diet plan immediately.

B. You may be dealing with serious / challenging health issues. This can help with avoiding too much "change."

C. Find that their body is less resilient and needs more time to adjust. If historically you've found it harder to transition to a new diet, this may be a better approach to help you "ease" into it.

D. Never been on a ketogenic diet, being fat-adapted is an adjustment for many.

E. Have limited experience with intermittent fasting (IF). Intermittent fasting can be challenging if you're used to constantly snacking. As you gain experience with the diet you'll likely realize it's more filling, but old habits can die hard and it's something to consider.

Although some proponents argue this diet may be relaxed and you can simply eat when and as much as you want, that is not optimal for your body. As your guide on this diet, we'll aim for optimal transition while giving ourselves room to adjust and land with what works best for you. Once adjusted to Carnivore you'll discover that reducing the timeframe of eating will have positive effects on hormones and your overall health goals.

F. If you're unfamiliar with macro tracking. I'm a HUGE fan of cultivating and approaching things with self-discipline. By tracking macros you will be able to best optimize your fat:protein ratio. You will be able to ensure you're in ketosis for optimal metabolic benefits and also learn your total caloric consumption, allowing you to more easily set and stick to goals around body composition change, weight gain and weight loss.

Here's a video I made on Carnivore Diet macro tracking. Watch the video and follow the steps. All the tools are low cost or free. The process is simple and will automatically savyour progress.

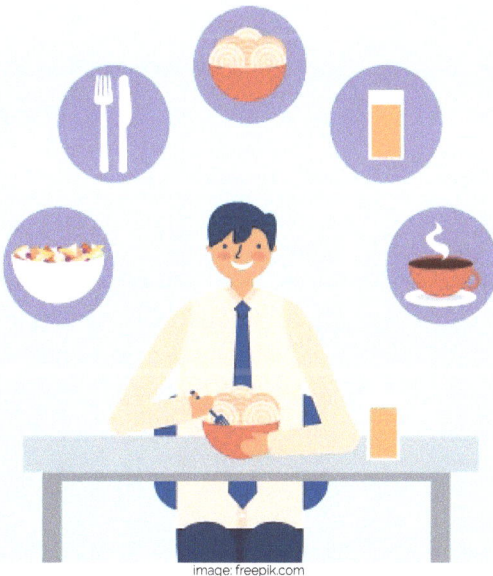

image: freepik.com

Eating Timeline

The Full On approach is fairly straightforward, while a Gradual approach can look a number of different ways. Let's break down a Gradual approach. In each week you'll slowly ratchet up your intake of Carnivore items while weaning down your elimination of plant foods.

Early on if you don't want to macro track that is okay. (Macro tracking is the process of weighing and counting protein and fat you eat and tracking them) Our biggest priority is getting off toxic foods and onto optimal eating. Once you've adjusted to 100% Carnivore you can introduce this. The other approach is simply do only Carnivore meals and start to gradually macro track progressively. I'll leave that decision up to you.

Each chart below lists off a suggested week of eating with the three meals for breakfast, lunch and dinner, Sunday through Saturday. Within the days / meals that you will be eating Carnivore I've placed a steak symbol. This does not mean you have to eat "steak" per se, but it does indicate this would be a meal absent of plant foods.

WEEK 1

	SUN	MON	TUE	WED	THU	FRI	SAT
BREAKFAST		🥩					
LUNCH			🥩			🥩	
DINNER							🥩

In our first week, we'll be working our way up to having **3 - 4 full Carnivore meals**, breakfast, lunch, or dinner. Eat as much whenever you want, not changing this pattern.

"I wouldn't be here if it weren't for a tremendous story that deeply impacted my life. This is the story of how I discovered the Carnivore Diet and how all of this came to be ".

WEEK 2

	SUN	MON	TUE	WED	THU	FRI	SAT
BREAKFAST		🫘	🫘			🫘	🫘
LUNCH		🫘	🫘			🫘	🫘
DINNER		🫘	🫘			🫘	🫘

By week two we're now on to 3-4 full Carnivore days. In week one you might've had steak and eggs for breakfast with a steak and a salad for lunch, and salmon for dinner. You'll now be eliminating the salad. (Yes this can be healthy, don't panic!) Outside your Carnivore days and meals you'll be consuming what you most are used to prior.

WEEK 3

	SUN	MON	TUE	WED	THU	FRI	SAT
BREAKFAST	🫘	🫘	🫘		🫘	🫘	🫘
LUNCH	🫘	🫘	🫘		🫘	🫘	🫘
DINNER	🫘	🫘	🫘		🫘	🫘	🫘

In week three, we're simply upping the days of Carnivore consumption. We'll go from 3-4 Carnivore days to 5-6 Carnivore days. The majority of your week will now be running on Carnivore days. You will have the occasional meal that includes plants and fruits but you'll be mostly Carnivore at this point. Consider sharing your progress by tagging yourself and your journey #karnivorekurt @karnivorekurt

WEEK 4

	SUN	MON	TUE	WED	THU	FRI	SAT
BREAKFAST							
LUNCH							
DINNER							

In your 4th and 5th weeks you'll now be full Carnivore for 1-2 weeks in a row. You'll start to narrow down the animal foods and focus largely on beef and fish. At this point you'll be going for stretches of 7-14 days without any plant molecules. The occasional event or slip-up may happen but you're likely almost exclusively Carnivore. At this point, if not already, you're likely to start seeing real improvements in how you feel along with any auto-immune / inflammation likely lowering.

WEEK 5

	SUN	MON	TUE	WED	THU	FRI	SAT
BREAKFAST							
LUNCH							
DINNER							

In the 5th week, *after roughly one month of transitioning, you're now full on Carnivore. At this point it's all about optimizing for micronutrients.* Start **introducing organ meats, specifically kidney and liver.** For many, these organs can have a stronger flavor. Preparing them in different ways can really help make them more palatable. I've created a video here on a Liver Jerky recipe which I've found is often easier to consume and travel with. I'd also suggest trying a small amount of ghee and salt (if you do okay with ghee) as another alternative.

Your gut and body should be fairly well adjusted, your fridge and cabinet are likely adjusted to support this diet as well and you're probably experiencing several of the benefits of mood, gut, sleep, strength and energy. Many of those benefits might have already been experienced in the weeks prior.

WEEK 6

	SUN	MON	TUE	WED	THU	FRI	SAT
BREAKFAST							
LUNCH							
DINNER							

We will start to remove all meats except beef, organs and high quality, clean fish. Pork and eggs tend to be harder to source in high quality. That often makes them more triggering for many people. We'll remove them so you can really see and feel the effect of the maximal experience of a total elimination diet Carnivore Diet. If you haven't yet, also remove all spices and seasoning. Salt, beef, fish and water are the optimal at this stage.

Note - We'll talk more about concerns around coffee and tea, for now you can keep those items if you really want. Try best to avoid creamers, sugars and syrups.

WEEK 7

	SUN	MON	TUE	WED	THU	FRI	SAT
BREAKFAST							
LUNCH							
DINNER							

Transition cooking methods to almost always lightly blanching all food. Consume fats in their raw form and limit the melted, rendered fat from butter or meat left in pans. This will remove PAHs (Polycyclic Aromatic Hydrocarbons) and HCAs (Heterocyclic Amines) and avoid gut issues caused by the rendered fats.

If you decide to intermittent fast or skip a meal here or there combine the food items. These graphics are here to show the consumption of the day. The timing and amounts will vary based on your strategy of when you feel best for eating.

Although the quantities in the studies were significantly higher than what one would be expected to eat, PAHs and HCAs are compounds that have been linked as causal in studies as carcinogenic. Additionally eating meats and fats in their rare form will preserve more nutritional value and help with improving nutritional absorption and keeping the gut at ease. After a week or two transition, you'll start to feel really energized.

Cooking can break chemical bonds and evaporate water soluble vitamins - B and vitamin C. Eating meat extremely rare and simply searing off the surface bacteria / pathogens will preserve the highest nutrient load for your body while removing the majority of potential food-borne contaminants. Always purchase your meat through a reputable source, keep frozen and consume promptly after thawing. If you don't like rare, that's okay. Just note you may want to pay closer attention to B and C water-soluble vitamin nutrient deficiencies. You may want to add more organs and shellfish down the line to compensate for the evaporation and damage from higher heat and longer cooks.

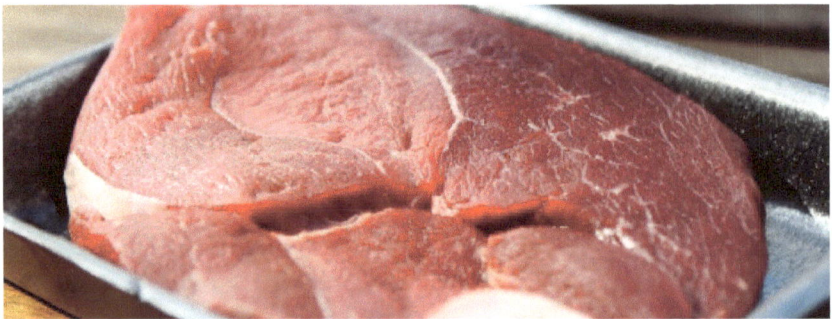

Image: freepik.com

Full Carnivore

It's suggested to do Carnivore for 60 days to allow the body to heal and recover. You've made it. This is the Promised Land where things truly magical can happen with health and vitality.

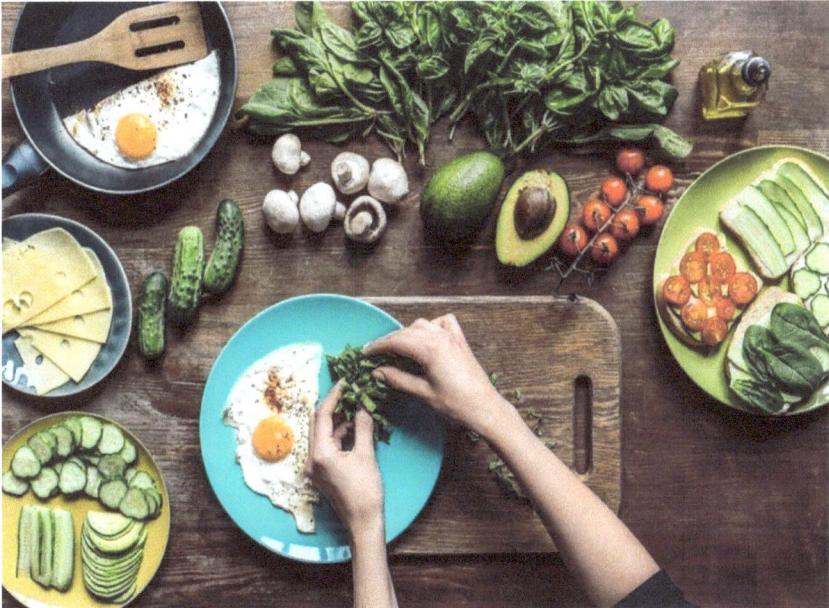

Image: Reintroducing different foods back in to see how one feels

Reintroduction

One of the most powerful components to this diet is how clear and in touch one becomes with their body. The amount of dietary noise is drastically eliminated when you're eating purely high quality carnivore. The smallest of additions and changes to your diet and regimen will be much more noticeable. Your sensitivity to feeling and realizing what throws you off will be substantially improved. I used to "tolerate" so many things. Now I realize how powerfully they impacted me in a negative way. I can easily tell if something isn't optimal for my body and diet.

— 14. TOXIC VS TOLERABLE —
PLANTS

One of the primary reasons to embark on this diet is to remove triggering foods; molecules that when added to our human biochemistry cause real disruptions and issues with our physiology.

Remember plants co-evolved with animals over millions of years and developed natural mechanisms to prevent predation. Plants have natural pesticides that can kill and seriously poison their predators. Keep in mind these two categories can vary from individual to individual. Some do better with certain food items while others have much more severe reactions.

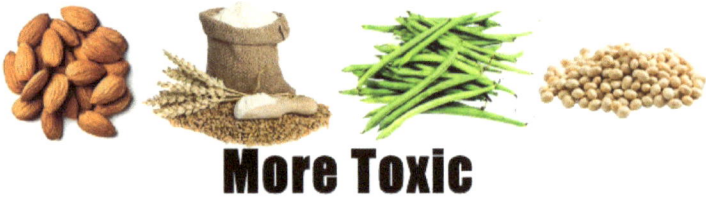

More Toxic

Image: More toxic plant foods

More Toxic

Seeds are the most heavily defended. Seeds, grains, nuts and beans contain digestive enzyme inhibitors, lectins, glutens, phytic acid and several xeno hormetic molecules. That's right, xeno hermetics are NOT good for you despite the billion dollar industries that sell and tout their benefits. Their net effect can be quite damaging.

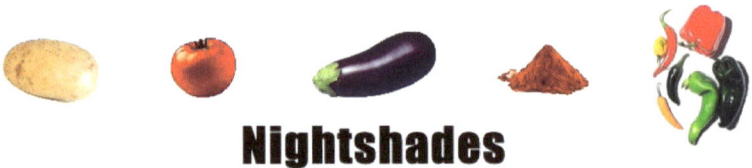

Nightshades

Image: Nightshades, some of the most triggering plant molecules

In addition nightshades: eggplant, goji berries, tomatoes (these all have elf shaped stems) are highly likely to cause immune reactions.

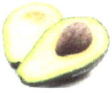

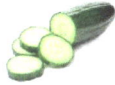

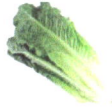

More tolerable

Image: More tolerable foods

More Tolerable

Avocado, cucumbers, lettuce, and olives as well as various squashes are actually foods that most will do better with. Remove skins and seeds when possible.

━━━ 15. NOSE TO TAIL ━━━

The term nose to tail refers to eating animal foods in their entirety. This means NOT eating just muscle meat, steaks and water. It means including parts of the animal less common, but dense in unique micronutrients not as prevalent in other parts.

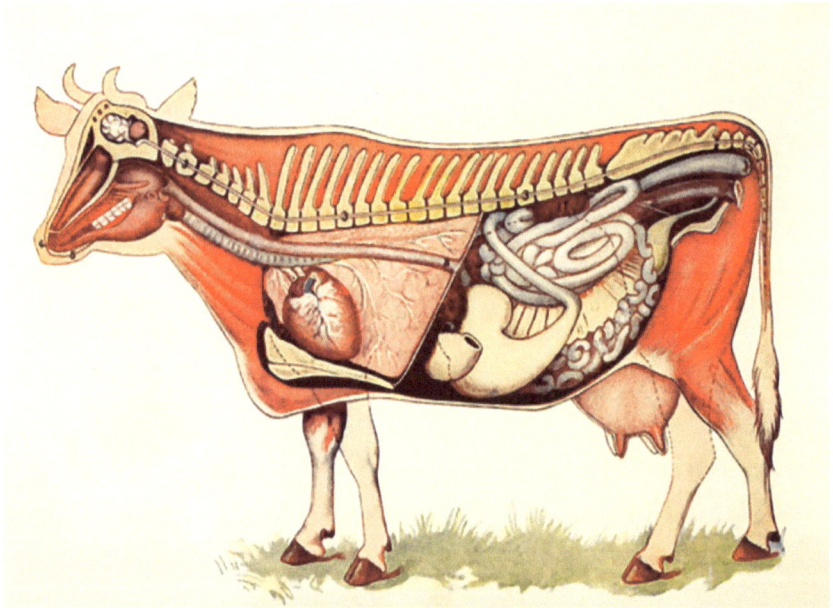

Image: Ruminant animal nose to tail

Organ meats and connective tissues are a key component here. *A nose to tail approach* ***must include liver and kidney****. Other organs may more easily be skipped but these two are essential to cover all micronutrients.* From my experience of nearly a 1,000 consecutive Carnivore meals, and researching the nutritional profile, liver and kidney pack the most punch in the best balance for most people.

Generally I steer people towards **grass fed beef** over lamb, pork or chicken. This is probably the closest ruminant animal to the ancestral megafaunal we consumed in large quantities during some of our greatest evolution to becoming human animals. High quality grass fed beef is one of the most tolerated foods for humans on the planet. It also provides one of the best nutritional profiles both from its muscle and organ meats. In fact, it gives us everything we need when we add in sunshine, and the minerals from high quality spring water.

Organs

Beef liver has an incredible profile of vitamins and minerals that are in the exact forms humans need. It is considered by many as one of, if not the most, nutrient dense food a human can consume.

	100g Beef Liver	500g Beef Steak	Total
Sodium	4%	20%	24%
Potassium	7%	45%	52%
Calcium	1%	5%	6%
Magnesium	5%	30%	35%
Phosphorous	46%	110%	156%
Chloride	4%	25%	29%
Iron	63	80%	63.8%
Zinc	47%	235%	282%
Copper	466%	30%	496%
Vitamin A	2200%	8%	2208%
Vitamin B1	23%	40%	63%
Vitamin B2	218%	65%	283%
Vitamin B3	112%	260%	372%
Vitamin B5	132%	25%	157%
Vitamin B6	60%	60%	120%
Vitamin B7	75%	15%	90%
Vitamin B9	60%	5%	65%
Vitamin B12	2000%	820%	2820%
Vitamin C	22%	0%	22%
Vitamin D	2%	9%	11%
Vitamin E	2%	20%	22%
Vitamin K2	127%	95%	222%

Image: Micronutrient content beef liver vs beef steak

Personally I experienced a bit of vitamin A toxicity while consuming ~ 4-5oz (110-140 grams) of raw beef liver daily for 2 months. After doing this, I started experiencing blurred vision, headaches and sinus pressure. When I discussed this with @CarnivoreMD, and did my own digging, I realized what was going on and cut it out for a week. After only 2-3 days, I started feeling much better. A week later I was almost back to normal. I usually hover around 155 lbs and consume around 2,600 calories daily. I now eat about 25-35 grams (1-2oz) of liver every 2-3 days.

That said, too much of a good thing can be a bad thing. Beef liver is exceptionally high in vitamin A and copper - both incredible nutrients, but ones that can be taken in excess if one is not careful. Because of these high amounts, I recommend most people consume beef liver 2-4/week, 2-4oz at a time depending on needs and a person's size. Most people can tolerate overconsumption of micronutrients for a while so unless you're consistently consuming at high quantities, this isn't something I would worry too much about.

Water soluble vitamins and minerals are generally less accumulated than fat soluble vitamins and nutrients such as vitamin A, D and E and K. This is why you see supplements with 10,000 times the daily value of B and C vitamins one needs. It's generally much safer and easier for the body to urinate out excess quantities of the water-soluble vitamins.

Beef kidney

Beef kidney has many key vitamins as well. But contains a lot less vitamin A. I usually consume 3-4 oz

	100g Beef Kidney	100g Beef Liver
Energy (kcal)	96 kcal	139 kcal
Fat	3.3 g	4 g
Carbohydrates	0.9 g	5 g
Protein	15.7 g	20 g
Water	78.9 g	1.3 g
Sodium	12%	16 mg
Potassium	6%	7%
Calcium	1%	1%
Magnesium	6%	5%
Phosphorous	35%	51%
Chloride	9%	4%
Sulfur	170 mg	240 mg
Iron	76%	56%
Zinc	24%	57%
Copper	35%	252%
Manganese	3%	7%
Flouride	5%	3%
Iodide	2%	7%
Vitamin A (Retinol)	37%	1700%
Vitamin B1	27%	25%
Vitamin B2	188%	240%
Vitamin B3	41%	98%
Vitamin B5	64%	122%
Vitamin B6	20%	42%
Vitamin B7	24%	100%
Vitamin B9	0%	55%
Vitamin B12	3100%	6500%
Vitamin C	11%	23%
Vitamin D	5%	9%
Vitamin E	2%	5%
Vitamin K2	0 ug	75 ug

Image: Beef kidney vs beef liver *note vitamin a and copper values consume 3-4 oz of beef kidney 4-5 days / week (skipping liver on those days). One of the reasons I really like kidney is because kidney contains a unique enzyme called diamine oxidase.

The section on allergies below will go into more detail on this topic, but know that this nutrient can help many people break up excess histamine build up in their body. Rather than take antihistamines, which suppress these critical neurotransmitters, you can fuel your body to properly monitor and break allergies down when they get excessive.

The vitamin content is a bit less drastic so I'm less concerned with over-doing a good thing and getting too much of any particular nutrient.

We'll talk more in the meal plans section, but the general approach I take right now is to consume the animal nose to tail and try and incorporate different elements of the cow regularly.

Some weeks I'll eat more steaks - sirloins, ribeyes and skirt steak, while other weeks I might be consuming mostly bone (broiled and then marrow scooped out), connective tissues and chuck cuts. I'll rotate the fat I add that accompanies these protein heavy items with beef suet (the fat around internal organs), beef fat, pork fat and lamb fat.

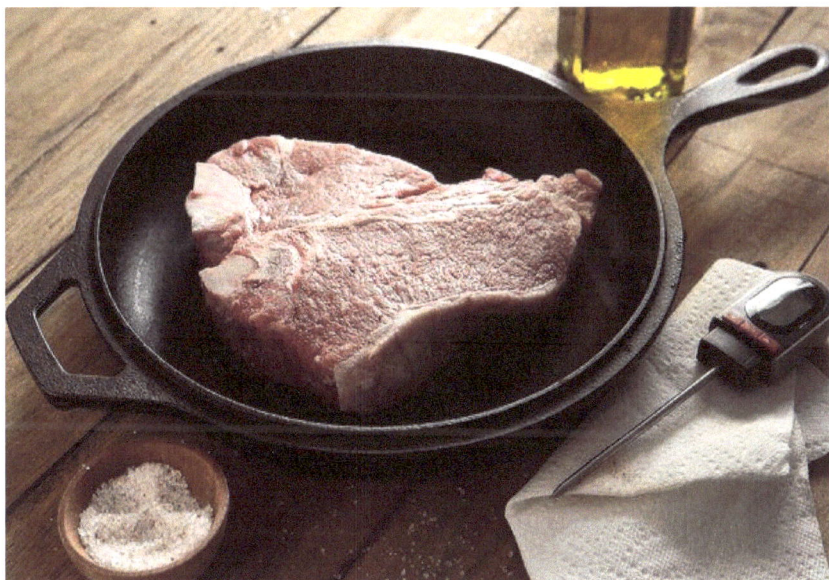

Image: Porterhouse steak in iron skillet

16. COOKING FOR OPTIMAL NUTRITION AND FEEL

Interestingly, cooking can have a surprisingly dramatic impact on how well you feel. It also changes the molecular structure of food depending on how you cook it. It took me a while to really figure this out, but what I share below will likely really help many of you and your gut. In this section, let's talk about a few approaches that have made a major impact on my Carnivore and overall nutrition experience.

Cookware

For cooking I recommend using a stainless steel pan. Ceramic or cast iron are close second options in terms of the most optimal for leaching chemicals into the food. [32] Non-stick teflon pans are no longer the rave and have serious issues.

Ghee for the Win!

For newer carnivores who are craving more flavor and variety, organic grass fed ghee (clarified butter) is usually my recommendation as the optimal choice for "cooking oil." Butter isn't bad but Ghee is usually safer for gut issues as it is lactose free and clarified. I often see people liberally adding these to their foods. If it works for you great. I've noticed hours later I will get gut pain and cramping and it's exactly from too much butter/ghee. Because of this I don't use that much (a teaspoon) to avoid larger quantities of melted down rendered cooking fats and oils.

In my personal experience and talking with many, these often trigger gut issues even for the adapted carnivores when consumed in larger quantities. It will vary from person to person and from the types of butter to ghee as to how well your gut does. You can find Ghee at any major health food store or online. It's quite easy to order and have shipped and stores for months at room temp.

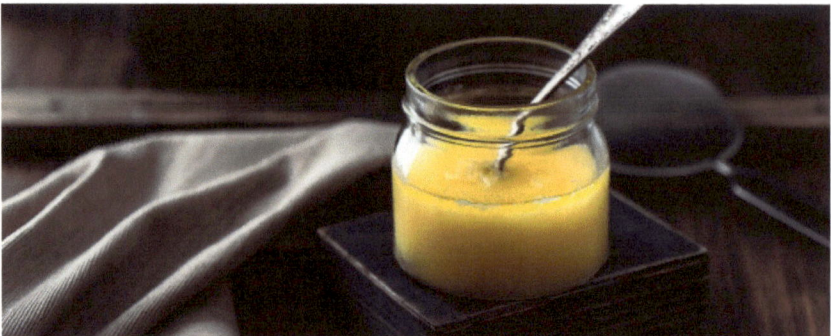

Image: http://livecrushoil.com/product/desi-cow-ghee/

Blanching

For those wanting to go a level further on the health side, I recommend blanching. Simply add 0.5-1" of water to the surface of the pan. Heat it up to medium and place the meat in the water. Blanching will limit HCAs and PAHs, compounds caused from burning and charring of the meat, both of which can stress your body.

I'm not a fan of sous-vide cooking methods because you're cooking in a plastic bag. Plastic is already in everything [33] and we know even the BPA-free versions can leach into the food and disrupt the body and your hormones.

Throw out your plastic water filters and bottles in exchange for glass or stainless steel. Yes, BPA-free plastics can leach into your water. *Sigh* even aluminum cans are lined with plastic. [34]

Ground Beef

If you're consuming ground beef you'll want to thoroughly cook it. Due to the process of grinding up the outer meat exposed to the inner portions, ground beef has a much higher chance of containing food-borne illnesses. Personally I rarely eat ground beef. I don't like having to cook it so much. It tends to liquify the fat more, again leading to potential gut issues and lowering the nutritional density. I prefer whole cuts in a less processed form. As you get more experience, you'll be able to find and track down better meat cuts.

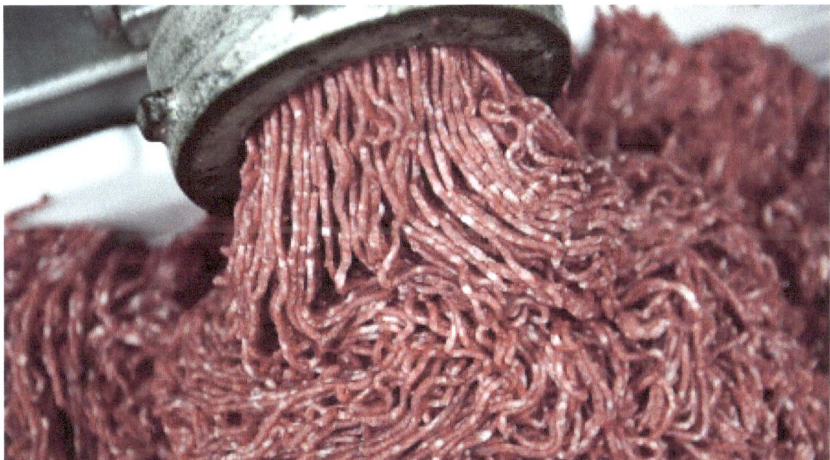

Image: https://www.cnbc.com/2019/04/12/cdc-suspects-ground-beef-is-the-source-of-recent-e-coli-outbreak.html

Going Raw Carnivore (Warning)

Some people go raw. I tried it out and did find it more satiating and ended up feeling more full eating a lower volume of food, but it was much less palatable. I noticed that I just didn't like eating raw meat nearly as much from a taste perspective and I had to be much more careful with the "freshness" and "quality." There may be some nutritional benefits in terms of further preserving water soluble vitamins (B,C), as well as proteins being less damaged from cooking.

If you're blanching the exterior and eating meat rare I think you're still preserving much of the nutritional profile, while substantially eliminating chances of capturing food-borne illnesses. *The only food I now eat raw is beef liver, largely due to how rich in vitamins and nutrients it is, I prefer to preserve its vitamins and nutrients as much as possible.*

Eating raw is not recommended, unless you're already an advanced Carnivore and are well adapted and in touch with the source of your food. The thinking is that the nutritional profile combined with our exceptionally high gut acidity is a powerful combination that can give you even more nutrients in a more bioavailable form. Cow sushi if you will.

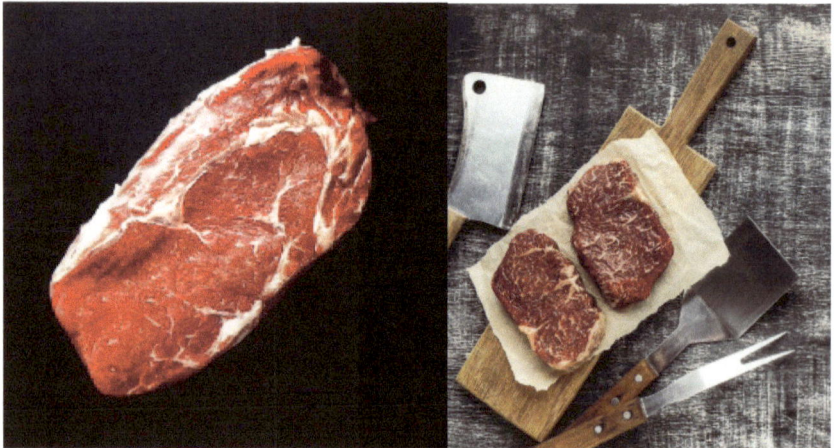

Image: freepik.com

Slow Cooks

I own a crock and instant pot. The food that comes out of these cooking contraptions **is delicious**. BUT, I find I usually struggle with the increased histamines slow cooks produce and more so the liquified fat that melts off the meat. (I discuss histamines at length in the section on allergies.) The melted fat is more likely to make its way through your intestines into your large intestine and colon unabsorbed. This can cause those regions to secrete more water in aiding the breakdown of food that would normally be absorbed in the stomach and small intestine prior to reaching it. When unabsorbed food meant for earlier parts of the gut passes towards the later digestive sections, and combines with water, this can cause diarrhea and other disease in the digestive system.

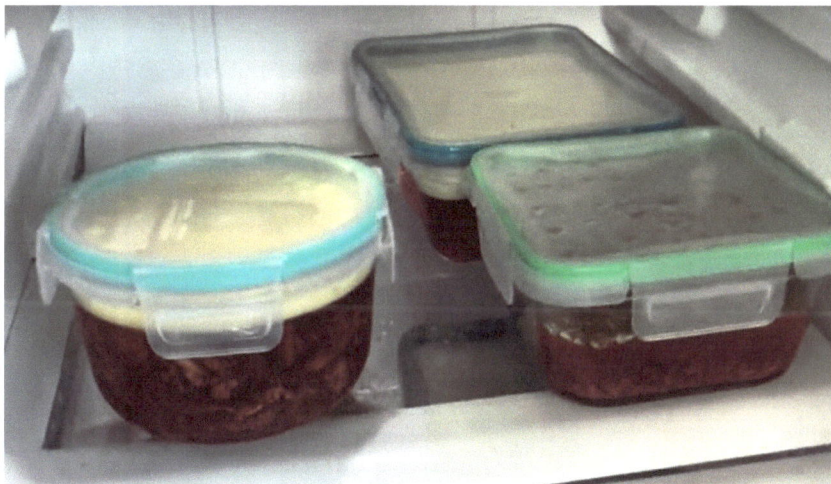

Image: Slow cooked broth solidified left and back right show thick fat layer, right front shows fat layer scraped off

Slow cooked bones and tendons now solidified into gelatin. Left circle glassware shows a thick layer of fat on top, you can see the right square in front has had that layer scraped off, making it much more tolerable.

One hack that helps with this is taking the whole slow cook, let it sit at room temp and then scraping off the fat that will float and solidify to the top. This will usually make that food much more tolerable to my gut, but it removes a lot of that great fat and fat soluble vitamins and minerals so it's a trade off.

On one hand you'll get valuable nutrient rich collagen and connective tissue much harder to obtain when regularly eating, but on the other hand it'll be void of fat so you'll have to pay attention to that. Ultimately I think it's valuable to make these types of things for the collagen and glycine you get. Just be careful as they can trigger histamine and gut issues if you consume too much and don't take heed to remove the rendered fats. (Some people will tolerate this much better than I do, so play with it and see how you do.)

This diet is fat heavy so we want to be getting lots of great quality fat ~ 70%+ of our calories to be more precise. A lot of nutrients are stored in the animal fat, something to keep in mind you're trading off with when scraping off the rendered slow-cooked fat.

Us Wellness - Grass Fed Beef Brisket

Serving Size : 3 oz ▾

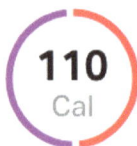

	0%	100%	100%
110 Cal	-- **Carbs**	**4g** Fat	**17g** Protein

Image: Macronutrients of grass fed beef brisket

Not to discourage you, but you'll need to account for the much lower caloric total when consuming slow-cooked foods where you remove the rendered fat. If for example you slow cook a grass fed brisket, you'll want to tweak the "volume" within your macro tracking app of the food, to try and adjust for the 0g of fat that now exist from the slow-cooking method.

these nuances around adjusting the macros are much more important with weight gain and weight loss goals. They are still valuable to build a habit and to help you better understand how much food you want, and need, to be eating.

To be clear, if I consume raw, unrendered, uncooked fat, it breaks down in the stomach and small intestine and is absorbed more consistently and easily by my body before it hits my large intestine and colon. But as soon as the fat is melted, there's a much higher chance I'm on the toilet with cramping and loose stools.

Consuming the Fat

This is a tricky one and I think one of the biggest challenges people have with adapting and really keeping to a Carnivore and Ketogenic type diet. Both are going to require ~ 70-80% fat intake and if you don't have a solid source of fat you're going to really struggle on this diet.

High quality egg yolks can be a great source of both fats and high quality micronutrients. But you really want to find high quality eggs. Vital Farms organic pastured eggs would be at the **bottom tier of quality** in my experience. You'll notice higher quality eggs often have richer, deeper orange egg yolks and (here's the real tell) **whites that are thicker, sticking to the yolk and more yellow** in color. This really indicates that the chickens have been outside getting sunlight on their feathers producing vitamin D. Personally I find the best egg sources are local farmer's markets and local co-ops that will buy from local farmers.

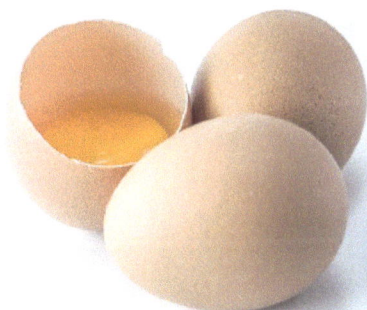

Image: freepik.com

At farmer's markets you can talk to the farmers and ask them direct questions about how they are raising their animals and what they are actually feeding them. Usually, though not always, the food items will be competitively priced at the markets as well. Interestingly, though egg yolks are more liquid in form - I have never had gut issues consuming 4-5 raw yolks in a sitting (I usually crack the eggs over my sink and sift out the yolks to eat raw). That said, they are in their native form and are around 75% fat, 25% protein.

Egg whites contain mostly protein and are nutritious. But due to the significantly higher vitamin and micronutrient content of the yolks, I prefer to limit the whites to assist with staying in line with my goal of maintaining a 70%+ fat intake. There's nothing innately wrong with consuming high quality whites, but I find I like the yolks for their vitamins and minerals and the added calories and protein from the whites can tip my macros out of balance for what I want. If you do consume eggs you will want to cook the whites to break down avidin, which can bind to biotin. Leave the yolks runny for maximal nutrition.

Raw Suet, Raw Tallow, Fat Trimmings

One of my biggest game-changers, in terms of gut stability and ease was when I was introduced to raw fat trimmings. Suet and tallow are all animal fats, but in particular I'm talking about what you get directly from the animal processor that is not melted and processed. Companies like EPIC brand carry rendered beef and bison tallow in jars which you can find at Whole Foods. But these are not in their raw form and in my experience, will cause gut issues.

The raw forms that have not been cooked on the other hand are incredibly tolerable to the gut. They break down slower and the body usually absorbs them quite well. You can source these items from local butcher shops, farmer's markets and online sources. All you've got to do is call around and go to the markets and ask the farmers. If they don't have those by default, it's as simple as putting in an order which they'll fill the next time they visit the market. This goes for kidney and liver as well - though liver can often be found in Whole Foods and other health food stores quite easily.

Bottom line, how you cook your food will vary and impact both the quality of nutrition as well as how well you digest it. Learning these nuances early in your Carnivore journey will help avoid a lot of pain and challenge while adapting and learning this way of eating.

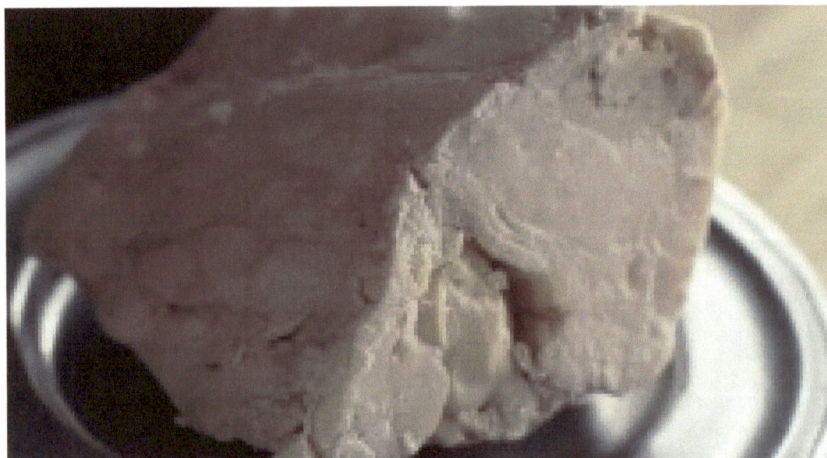

https://savoringthepast.net/2013/01/21/suet-part-two-what-it-is-what-it-isnt-and-what-to-look-for/

17. GRASS FED VS. GRAIN-FED

Which is better and why? Let's take a closer look at how the animals are typically raised and dive into their life cycle and what they're usually fed to see how this shakes out.

Regulations / Confusion Grain-Fed

All calves (baby cows) start off drinking cow's milk. After a few months they start to feed on forage and shrubs near their birthplace. Early life for grain vs grass fed cattle is similar.

These cattle are fed by their mothers and stay off pasture until they reach 650-750lbs. They're then moved to a feedlot of concentrated feed, typically grain, corn, soy and cereals. The young cow will feed for 3-4 months and fatten up to 1,200lbs to increase size and yield farmers can get. Often they can be kept in close quarters and fed antibiotics due to their reduced immune system and higher susceptibility of illness. It can be a brutal picture.

Grass Fed

These cows feed on grass the entirety of their lives. The USDA requires four signed documents to verify this diet. The guidelines are quite strict and most feel they are fairly robust to keep farmer's honest.

Lifetime / Cost

Grain-fed cattle typically are processed ~ 15 months, while grass fed take significantly longer, 20-24 months to reach maturity. This inherently costs more, keeping and raising cattle for longer periods of time.

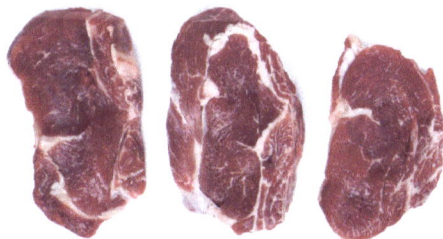

Image: freepik.com

Organic designations can be included in beef and they follow the same regulations of other organic foods.

Taste

Grain-fed cattle are often preferred due to their much higher marbling and fat content. Their meat is more tender, marbled and less "gamey" in taste and connective tissue.

Nutrition comparison

Studies are limited on the nutritional comparisons, but Alpha Tocopherol (Vitamin E), Beta Carotene and Ascorbic Acid (Vitamin C, more on this later) all appear more abundant in grass fed beef.

Table 1
Antioxidant vitamin levels in fresh beef

Treatment	α-tocopherol (µg/g)	β-carotene (µg/g)	Ascorbic acid (µg/g)
Grain	1.50 ± 0.73a	0.06 ± 0.03a	15.92 ± 3.48a
Grain + E	1.76 ± 0.97a	0.05 ± 0.01a	17.39 ± 4.29a
Pasture	3.08 ± 0.45b	0.45 ± 0.21b	25.30 ± 10.23b
Pasture + E	3.91 ± 0.74b	0.63 ± 0.27b	21.98 ± 5.11b

Means ($n = 10$ for each treatment) and standard deviation are indicated. Different letters within the same column differ ($P < 0.05$).

Image Source: Meat Science PubMed

Toxins

This one is tricky, but it's worth visiting. Like the nutrients listed above, the profile of toxins is a bit limited. We do know that animals can absorb what they eat and that can be passed on to those who eat the animals.

Pesticides and other chemicals are typically found in much higher concentrations within the feed of grains, but are not found in the grass and fields. Chemicals such as glyphosate (round-up), linked with leaky gut and cancer, and atrazine, which is a hormone disruptor, are much more likely to occur in grain-fed cattle due to their concentration in their feeds vs. grass fed.

Antibiotics and Hormones

Several antibiotics and hormones have been approved to treat sick cattle by the FDA. Some have concerns that injecting animals in order to maintain health and boost yield could lead to higher levels of these in the meat consumed by humans. Studies conducted thus far have suggested that we should not be concerned. The levels tested in such animals are far less than we produce in our human bodies. [22] We probably need more research, but if you have a choice, I'd opt for the grass fed. Antibiotics and hormones alone are probably not necessarily concerning.

Many of the hormones tend to be stored in the fats, so if this is of concern, opt for organic, grass fed fats vs grain-fed grain-finished.

Conjugated Linoleic Acid (CLA)

CLA is a unique type of trans fat found largely in the guts of ruminant animals, especially beef. It's been shown to protect against mammary cancer, aid in weight loss, body composition, improve insulin sensitivity and guess what? It is stored in much greater quantities in the fats of grass fed versus grain-fed cattle.

Studies have shown mixed outcomes when looking at CLA. We know some linoleic acid is needed, but how much is still unknown and how much more valuable conjugated is still being discovered. The overall consensus is that this nutrient may contain unique health benefits to support longevity and weight loss in humans.

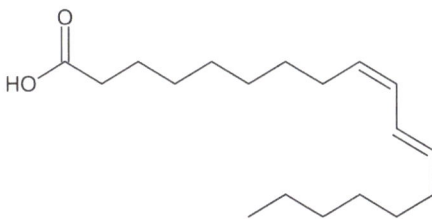

image: an example of conjugated linoleic acid

Environmental Impact

Grass fed crushes grain-fed here. Grass fed cattle produce less methane when eating their natural diet. They consume and require less toxic and environmentally damaging mono-crop grains (corn and soy), taking in less pesticides and need less antibiotics. Perhaps even more importantly, they protect and nurture the soil through their herd activities of defecating and urinating on the soil while stampeding it. They sequester their carbon and help recycle the lifecycle of carbon emissions[29].

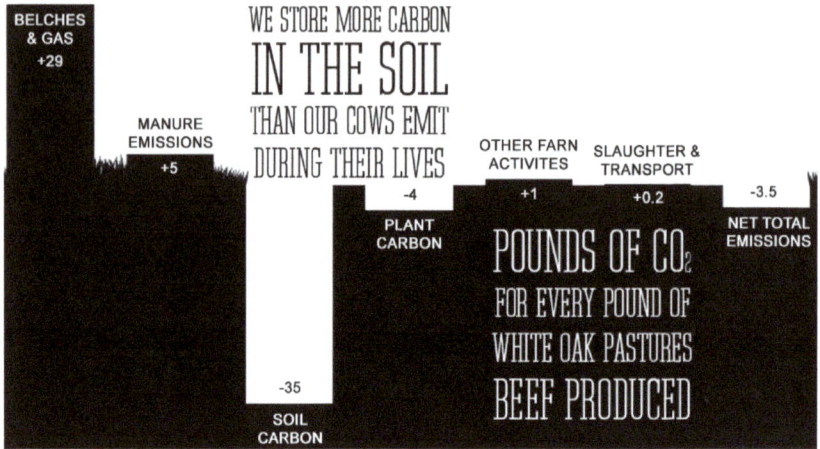

Image Source: Whiteoakpastures.com

Where Toxins Exist

Let's look at where in the animals different nutrition is stored. From there we can decide what might be worth investing, more toward grass fed or if it even matters all that much.

Fat & Organs

The majority of nutrition, omega-3 vs omega-6 fatty acids, Conjugated Linoleic Acid (CLA), fat-soluble vitamins (A, D & E) as well as the things we don't want: toxins, hormones and antibiotics are stored in the animal fat and organs. Additionally, I've found the cost of these items to be roughly the same, whether we go grain or grass fed. Because of this, I highly recommend sourcing all fat and organs from ONLY grass fed animals.

Muscle Meat

Steaks (muscle meat) largely store protein, minerals and water-soluble vitamins. Most muscle meat is lean, but it varies as grain-fed animals store more fats throughout their muscle as well. Think grass fed versus grain-fed ribeyes. The fat content can be 20-30% difference between the two.

Just like a human being that's sick and diabetic, continually feeding on processed sugars vs. someone that is out walking around and eating a more wholesome natural diet, you'd see a substantial difference in their body fat composition.

My recommendation for these cuts is to use your judgement. Don't let good become the enemy of great. Grain-fed cuts are still a good dietary choice if you're on a budget and that's all you can find and/or afford. Just do your best to try and avoid consuming higher quantities of grain-fed fats from these types of meats. Fattier cuts such as: ribeyes and strip steak usually have larger fat caps. (Areas of fat stores) Since potential toxins and hormones are stored in animal fat I would suggest sourcing these cuts only as grass-fed.

Overall, if you can afford grass fed cuts go for it! It's much better for the environment and animals. It will have a slight edge on nutrition, and you'll be voting with your dollar and supporting the planet. If you can't, grain-fed is still a great option for purchasing the leaner muscle meats. Most of the benefits between Grass fed vs Grain-fed actually show up in the animal fats, which won't matter much on cost, so go for grass fed on those.

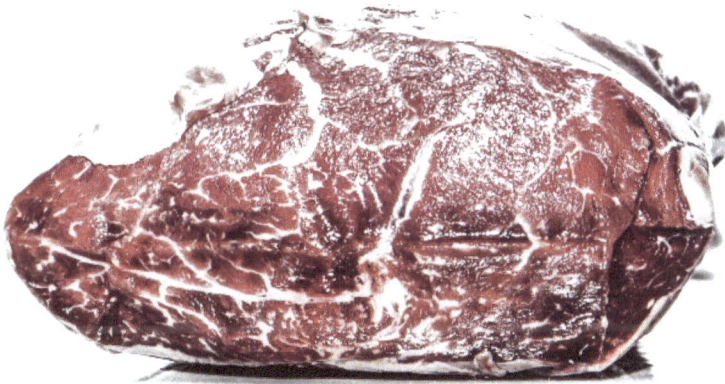

image: freepik.com

18. KIDNEY AND JOINT HEALTH

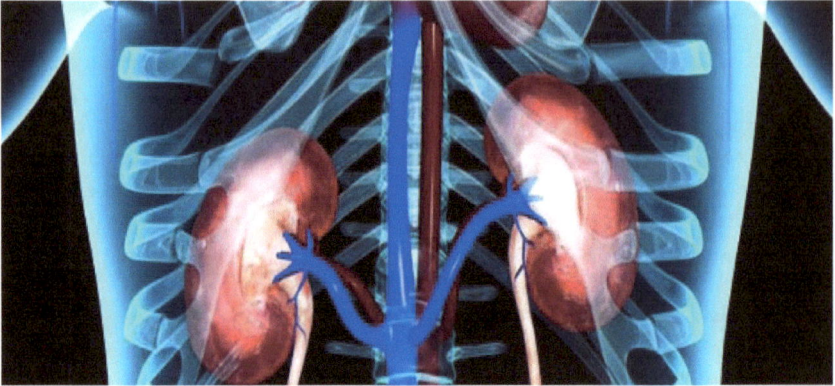

Image: Kidneys in human body

"Won't all this protein harm my health? My kidneys will most certainly fail and along with that accrue gout in my joints from all this uric acid build up!" This is a common misconception people have when they first learn about the Carnivore Diet.

One in nine US adults meet the requirements of having a decreased glomerular filtration rate (GFR), one of the primary risk factors for reduced kidney (renal) function, potentially leading to Chronic Kidney Disease (CKD). But when we look at the data, there is no link between protein consumption and CKD. [35] [43] [44]

Back in the 1920s we learned through dog models there was a relationship between increased protein intake and elevated rates of creatinine and urea excretion. Renal blood flow and GFR were also increased.

When we test for renal failure and CKD we look at protein, specifically albumin to see if the kidneys are properly recycling that protein back into the body, or if it's being peed out in larger trace amounts than should otherwise flow from healthy kidneys. Failing kidneys fail to filter this out of urine and hence we see protein in urine with folks who have failing kidneys. This leads many to believe it's the protein consumption causing kidneys to fail. Not so fast!

To the public the message drawn from this observation is that high protein diets "overwork" the kidneys and may negatively impact function over time leading to disease. But having protein in your urine doesn't necessarily mean that consuming protein is what caused it. You can see why this might be a bit misleading.

While it is true that consuming more protein can increase the GFR of our kidneys, if your kidneys are healthy and in working order, with no signs of pre-existing failure, there are plenty of cases of extremely healthy kidney function in high protein consuming athletes.

Low GFR (filtration rate) or elevated creatinine (a by-product of creatine) may be signs of kidney failure. Elevated levels of BUN (blood urea nitrogen levels) are NOT, they are simply indicators that you have higher levels of urea nitrogen from higher levels of protein being broken down by the body. This in and of itself is not a bad thing, but simply a function of your system taking in more protein and breaking it down in a healthy way.

I'll just add that a well constructed ketogenic Carnivore Diet requires no more protein than most other paleo / or even plant based diets supporting a healthy individual. We're talking 20-30% of dietary calories equallying protein.

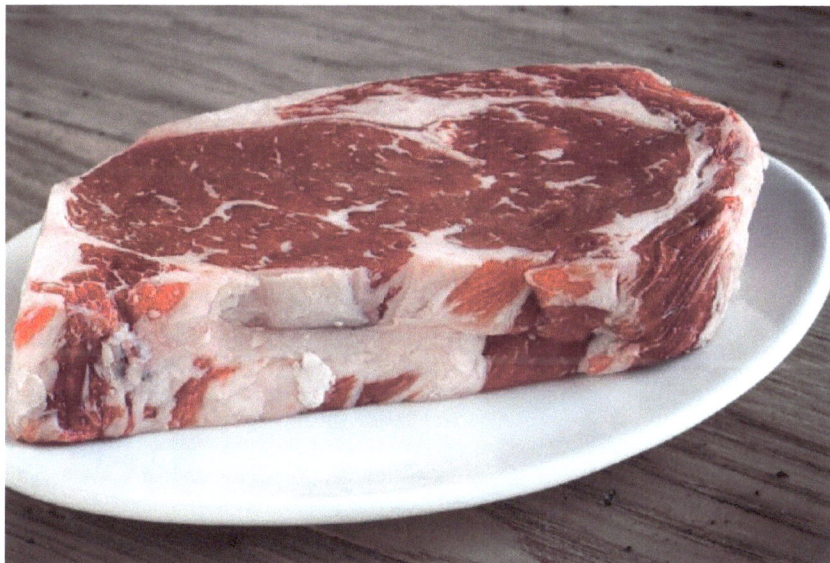

Image: freepik.com

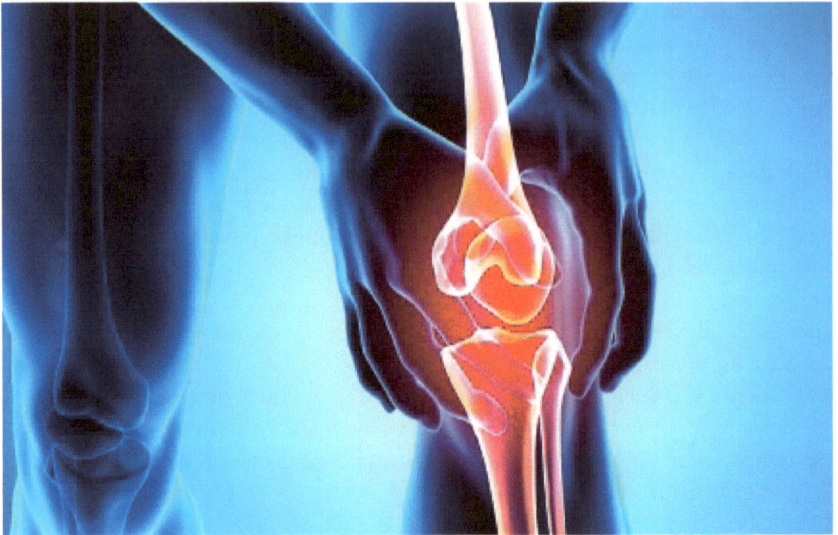

Image: Knee joint

Joint Health

Joint health isn't necessarily tied to kidneys, but it often can be. Gout is a condition of uric acid build up in the body. Uric acid is typically removed via the kidneys through urine, but when the kidneys don't function properly the body can get overloaded. Uric acid then forms and builds up in the joint areas and can cause painful arthritis.

That said, many of the success stories around crippling joint pain and arthritis are some of the most common things we see treated with the Carnivore Diet.[36] Bouts of chronic arthritis, inflammation, after living with for years of individuals' lives seem to quickly and miraculously cure and not return. I suspect the lowering of inflammatory omega-6 fats found largely in plant molecules combined with lack of auto-immune, inflammatory, gut membrane rupturing molecules is a bigger factor here. That combined with the powerful (almost exclusively found in animals) omega-3 anti-inflammatory fatty acid is much more likely a plausible explanation for this.

To close out this section I'll share my personal labs on kidney data for 90% red meat 13 months on Carnivore Diet. A few notes when reviewing these labs. My weight fluctuates between 154-158lbs most days, and I am usually around 9% body fat. I'm consuming 150 grams / protein / day, roughly 30% of my calories come from protein, 70% from fat.

Results (Non-Cardiometabolic)

Test Name	Current Result		Reference Range	Units	Lab
	In Range	Out of Range			
eGFR, Non-African descent	110		>60	mL/min/ 1.73 m²	Z4M
eGFR, African descent	128		>60	mL/min/ 1.73 m²	Z4M
BUN (Blood Urea Nitrogen)	16		8-23	mg/dL	Z4M
Creatinine	0.89		0.72-1.30	mg/dL	Z4M
BUN/Creatinine Ratio	Not Applicable		6-22	calc	Z4M
Albumin	4.1		3.5-5.5	g/dL	Z4M

Image: Kurt's renal (kidney health) lab results Nov 2019 one year on Carnivore

───── 19. ALLERGIES AND ─────
HISTAMINES

50 million Americans suffer from symptoms of allergies every year. [37] *Antihistamines are all the rave, but there's a vicious, uninformed side effect to taking these synthetic pharmaceuticals.* Histamine is actually a **neurotransmitter** in the human body that plays a key role in our immune function and alertness. Antihistamines work by binding to your body's receptors - essentially numbing your body's receptors to histamine.

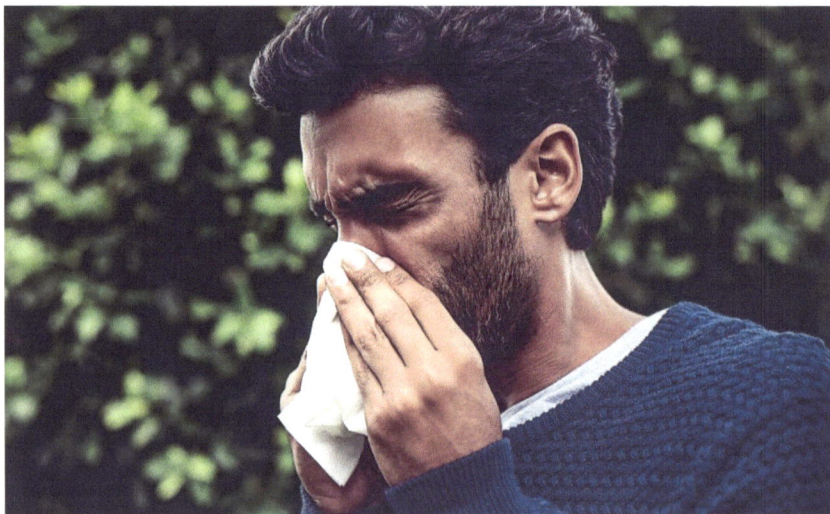
Image: Sinus congestion from allergies

While they can reduce the activity of allergic symptoms, they can also inhibit the activity in the learning centers of the brain and immune system. Antihistamine use has been directly linked with memory loss, in some cases **permanent memory loss**. Additionally they can impair cognitive performance. Not good. [55]

Rather than use a synthetic compound to numb your body's receptors and powerful system that aids in defenses and alertness, why not remove what's triggering this in the first place?

One of the largest sources of allergens for humans is diet. They are eating **high histamine foods** [38], foods that are triggering allergic reactions within the body. There are several foods that can be liberating of histamines and blocking of histamine enzymes that break down excess histamine.

When you think about it, allergic reactions to our environment outside us are just like allergic reactions to the foods we put inside us. There's a whole lot of exposure to toxins and reactions going on within the gut we just don't see. As a society we've become so accepting of eating and drinking foods, despite the impact they have on our biochemistry. It's crazy!

Antihistamines

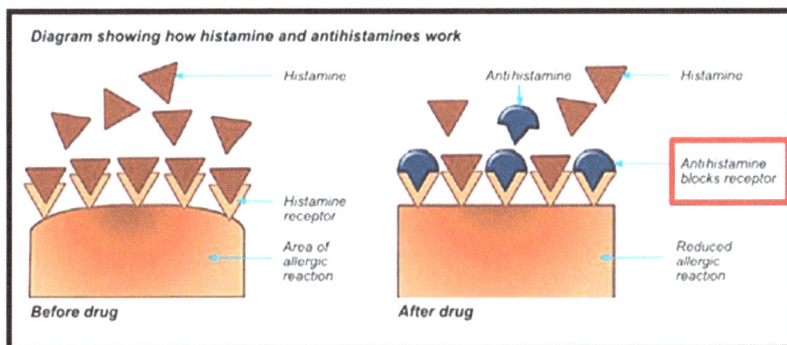

Image: Diagram of histamine antihistamine molecular interaction

The Carnivore diet can really help one avoid many of these food items, but it's still quite easy to be Carnivore and take in significant amounts of histamine. In particular canned foods, fermented foods, matured cheeses, smoked meats, cracklings, rinds, sausage, salami and bacon, as well as some shellfish, can be loaded with histamines. (Graphics below for reference)

These items tend to build up histamine levels in your body and almost always will be high in histamine. Additionally slow cooking meats builds up their histamine load! *Switch to a pressure cooker when possible, as cooking time can be a large factor in histamine build up.*

As your body gets exposed to more and more histamine triggering molecules your histamine load builds up. Usually there's a process when the body is able to clear out the build up, but if that's not occuring, one can get overloaded and experience severe symptoms and limitations.

These are liberators known to release more histamine from foods: Critic fruits, cocoa, chocolate, nuts, papaya, beans and pulses, tomatoes, wheat germ all contribute to histamine build up.

Foods to Avoid if You Are Histamine Intolerant

Histamine-Rich Foods

Fermented Alcoholic Beverages,
Fermented Foods: Sauerkraut, Vinegar, Soy Sauce, Kefir,
Yogurt, Kombucha, etc.
Vinegar-containing Foods: Pickles, Mayonnaise, Olives
Cured Meats: Bacon, Salami, Pepperoni, Luncheon Meats and Hot Dogs
Soured Foods: Sour Cream, Sour Milk, Buttermilk, Soured Bread, etc.
Dried Fruit: Apricots, Prunes, Dates, Figs, Raisins
Most Citrus Fruits
Aged Cheese Including Goat Cheese
Nuts: Walnuts, Cashews, and Peanuts
Vegetables: Avocados, Eggplant, Spinach, and Tomatoes
Smoked Fish and Certain Species of Fish: Mackerel, Mahi-Mahi, Tuna,
Anchovies, Sardines

Histamine-Releasing Foods

Alcohol
Avocados
Bananas
Chocolate
Cow's Milk
Nuts
Papaya
Pineapple
Shellfish
Strawberries
Tomatoes
Wheat Germ
Many Artificial Preservatives and Dyes

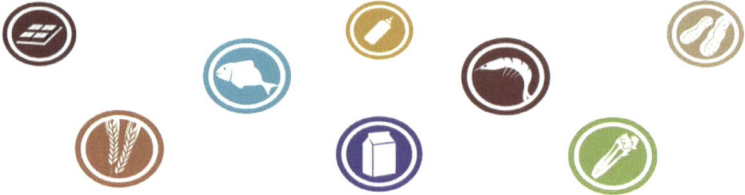

Image: Diagram of histamine antihistamine molecular interaction

High Histamine Foods:

Fresh foods (think fresh meats) are generally lower in histamine. Food items with a longer shelf life can be significantly higher: canned / fermented foods, alcohol, matured cheeses, smoked meats, salami, sausage, ham, bacon, and *sigh* of my old time favorites, smoked salmon. Shellfish, nuts, walnuts and cashews, vinegar, ready meals and salty snacks all fall into this category as well.

Diamine Oxidase (DAO):

Your body naturally produces and breaks down excess histamine using two enzymes, histamine-N-methyltransferase (HNMT) and Diamine Oxidase (DAO). Diamine Oxidase is the primary enzyme the body uses to break down histamine from food. Alcohol, black tea, energy drinks, green and maté teas all inhibit this enzyme.

Your kidneys produce this enzyme. Ironically eating kidney meat is an excellent source to boost levels of DAO. (Personally I eat 2-4 oz of raw beef kidney, 3-4x / week)

Fresh meats are low in histamine. The Carnivore diet can be very low in histamines when you avoid processed meats and focus on whole fresh meats. It can limit liberators and inhibitors; you'll have less production and levels of histamine triggering allergic symptoms in your body, hence reducing allergies from their SOURCE, without side effects of memory and alertness being compromised.

20. FIBER AND GUT HEALTH

Fiber has been promoted as the end all be all for human gut health. People are led to believe **if you don't consume fiber** you'll be more blocked up than a Calcutta sewer. Ironically, since I removed fiber from my diet, I've never felt better from a gut, digestion and bowel functioning perspective. Whenever I consume something highly fibrous, I usually experience the opposite; bloating, cramping and, well you get the idea. Let's get a bit scientific in this section because there's just so much noise on the value, the "studies" with context, there's so much nuance.

I get at least a dozen studies / week passed my way with conflicting "evidence" on eating Carnivore; how "dangerous" it is, how my gut is going to be loaded with cancer. I used to dive into all of them. Now I look very closely at the subject end points, as well as the context. When talking about fiber we have to be careful to consider the "benefits" claimed to slow down a diet. You'll learn in the section below on vitamin C, your body is a unique system that is likely shifting based on what method you run on. For me it's often more valuable to question biology and biochemistry. Below we'll look at some studies and then do exactly that.

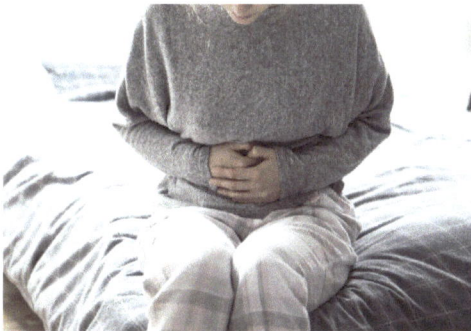

Image: freepik.com

A study that tracked 63 participants over the course of 2 years found that removing or reducing fiber was actually what improved bowel movements and their frequencies. [39] Another study [40] showed increased risk of diverticulosis that increased with consumption of fiber, it actually increases. Studies such as these support removing fiber resulting in improving digestive issues. Why would this be the case though?

Of course we can find counter "studies", but do we have controlled ones? The ones I found relied on participant questionnaires (they should be called "surveys"), excluding other healthy user bias and lifestyle factors. Studies like this one [41] make bold claims based on a lot of data that is arguably not reliable. Can you tell me what you ate, smoked, drank and did all last week with perfect accuracy?

Ancestry and Biology

Let's look at fiber and how it fits into ancestry as well as the biology of both humans and animals who consume it. Fiber is the insoluble, indigestible parts of plants. Think of the connective tissue that goes through a plant's leaves. The tough to break down, connective materials in plants. Humans get almost no calories from fiber.

High Fiber Eaters

Let's look at a couple of examples of "high" fiber diets in nature today.
Our gorilla ancestors today spend half their day chomping on leaves (highly fibrous portions of plants) to fill their much larger (football-sized) cecums and massive protruding guts. From that they're able to allow it to ferment in their gut into fats their body's can then utilize.

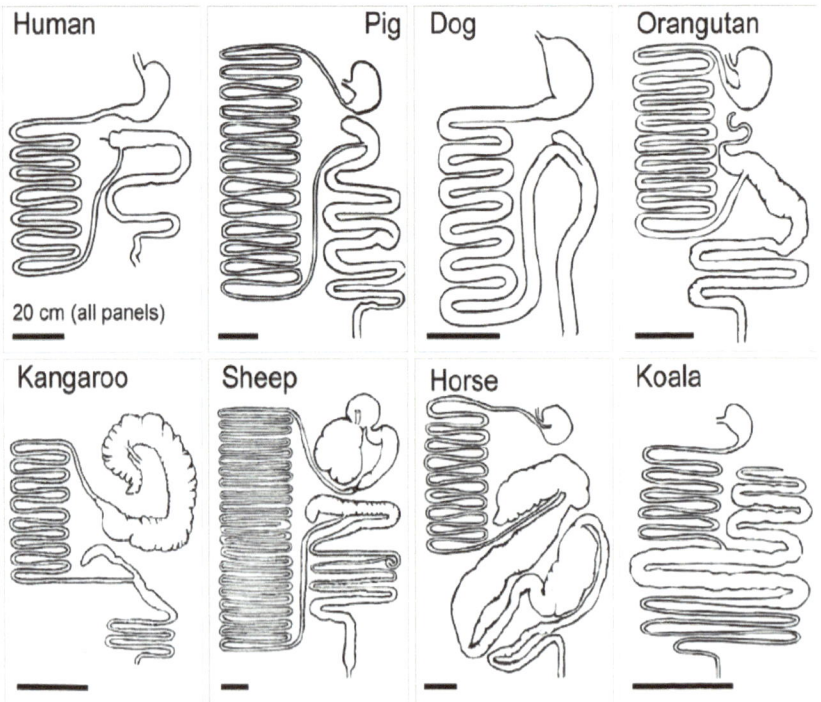

Image source: https://journals.plos.org/plosone/article?id=10.1371/journal.pone.0134116

Ruminant animals, cattle, sheep, goats, elk and deer all contain a digestive system much different than ours. It actually contains 4 compartments instead of a single stomach. They're uniquely built to handle many of the plant foods other animals cannot consume. Truly a unique and wonderful creation on this planet.

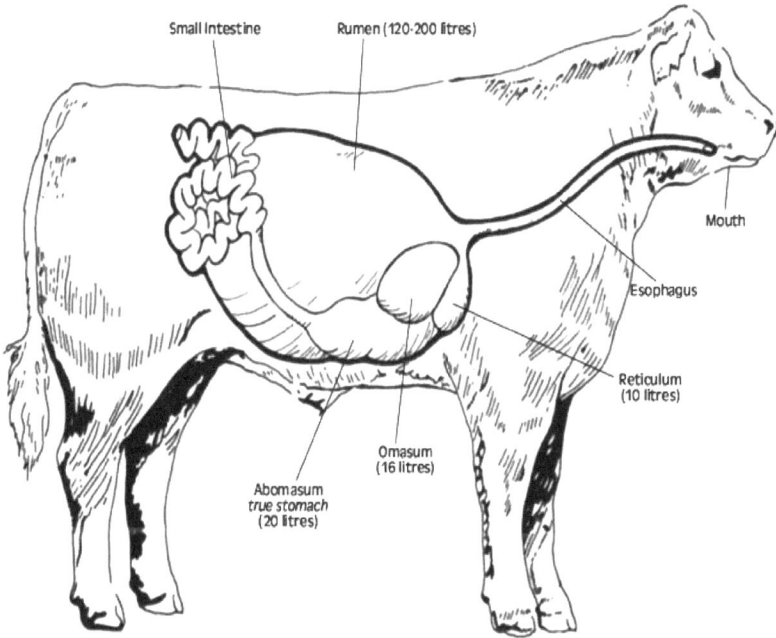

Small Intestine   Rumen (120-200 litres)

Mouth

Esophagus

Reticulum
(10 litres)

Omasum
(16 litres)

Abomasum
true stomach
(20 litres)

Image source: https://journals.plos.org/plosone/article?id=10.1371/journal.pone.0134116

Modern cattle spend 6 hours / day chewing up grass to consume up to 90 lbs of food / day. All this food goes into a rumen (50 gallon) first stomach section. Then they then puke it back up into their mouth and chew this regurgitated "crud" another 8 hours before sending it to their Osmasum to squeeze out the moisture before making its way to the abomasum where it mixes with digestive juices and makes it way to the intestine to be absorbed.

The high quantity of fiber from these diets is fermented in herbivores' guts and a huge place where that happens is in the colon. Humans have significantly smaller colons than our ancestor primates. [61]

Human guts don't look like those of ruminant animals or gorilla ancestors. We don't spend 8 hours chomping on and breaking down leaves and we don't have the volume of gut size to allow all this initially indigestible material to ferment into the nutrients.

The majority of research comes from epidemiological studies linking consumption of fiber-rich fruits and vegetables with lowered risks of obesity, heart disease and cancer, particularly colon cancer.

Keep in mind there are also billions of dollars in products every year going out on grocery shelves promoting their healthful fiber rich-ness. Yet randomized controlled trials tested in labs with consistent diets have not shown these protective effects to hold up. In some cases (more shared in the above referenced studies) we see the removal of fiber benefiting individuals. [62]

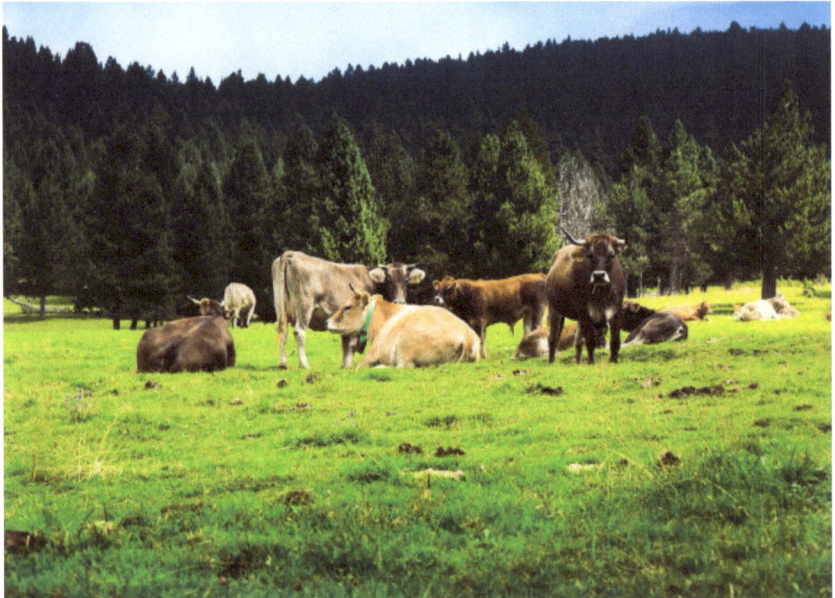

image.freepik.com

Gut Health

A discussion about the Carnivore Diet and fiber wouldn't be complete without going into gut health.

The human gut contains roughly 75% of all our immune cells. It is the second most concentrated area of neurons, housing more than 100M. The vagus nerve connects your mind/brain to your gut directly. When people say you have a "gut" feeling, they're not lying, you actually can feel what you eat.

Having gut issues isn't about a simple stomach problem. It feeds into your brain and mood. Your gut is a major area of entry for pathogens and diseases. Trillions of bacteria live in your gut and make up what's called the microbiome. After being broken down in the stomach, food passes to the small intestine. 90% of your nutrients are absorbed here. Arguably even more when consuming a diet high in animal foods.

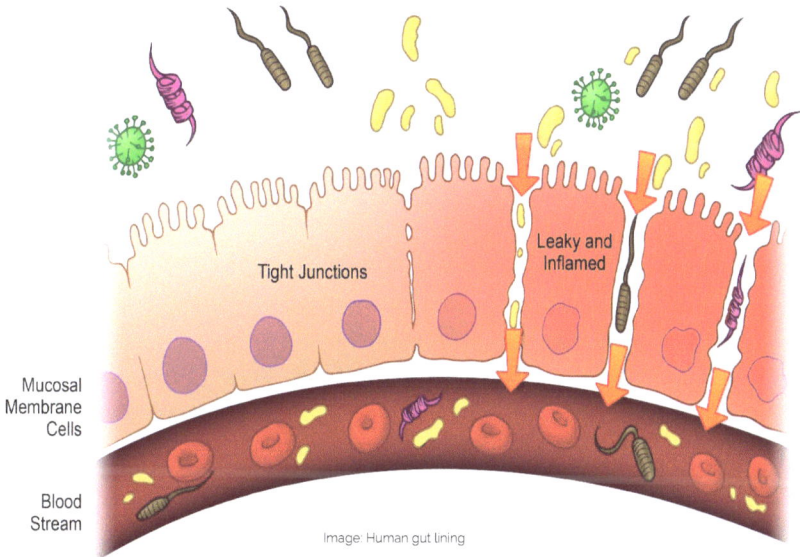

Image: Human gut lining

The small intestine's layer where it absorbs these nutrients is extremely delicate with thin, single cells of mucous linked together by proteins. This is the only layer separating what you eat from your bloodstream and your immune system is on guard to identify and attack any pathogens attempting to pass through.

When you eat foods that throw this system out of whack you can create dysbiosis and can even puncture the lining causing "leaky gut." Inflammation is a major trigger of penetrating this lining. When you consume foods that create inflammation and elevate this, your gut can struggle to stay on track and it can cause a whole slew of issues.

Removing inflaming foods that lead to disease within my own gut is one of the main reasons I feel as though this way of eating greatly improved my mood and anxiety.

Below is a list to consider adding to memory which helps outline the different plant groups, their defence chemistry and the effect it can have on human biochemistry.

Plant Group	Chemical	Effect
Almonds, beans, cherries, lesser extent corn, lima, peaches, tapioca	Cyanogenic glycosides	• Activated on bite • Release Neurotoxins • Block cellular respiration
Beans, legumes, lentils, peanuts, peas, wheat (WGA), zucchini	Lectins & saponins	• WGA causes leaky guts • Inflammation
Black tea, chocolate, grains, nuts, soy, spinach	Oxalates	• Reduces calcium and magnesium absorption • Kidney stones • May play a role in autism
Carrots, celery, limes, wild parsnip	Photosensitizers	• Make animals sensitive to light • Blistering and lesions
Chocolate, coffee, legumes, vinegar, wine	Phenolics & Tannins	• Zinc and iron deficiency
Citric, lemon, lemongrass, pepper	Terpenoids	• Volatile oils that can be highly toxic
Cruciferous Veggies: Aragula, broccoli, brussels sprouts, cauliflower	Sulforaphane	• Induces cancer cell death • Poisons mitochondria, kills healthy cells, generates reactivve oxygen species
Grains, legumes, nuts skin, stevia	Alpha-amylase inhibitor	• Dysbiosis, which can lead to leaky gut
Grains, nuts, potatoes, seeds	Phytics Acid	• Reduces mineral absorption, like zinc, iron and calcium
Nightshades: Eggplant, potatoes, tomatoes	Alkaloids	• Damages carb and fat metabolism • Damages DNA Repair • Damages nerve transmission

@karnivorekurt

The Carnivore Diet often works very well to improve gut issues through eliminating and reducing this constant bombardment of inflaming and breaking within the gut barrier.

Food intolerances vary by person but often include things such as:

- FODMAP foods
- Gluten, Lectins
- Phytic acid, Grains
- Refined Sugars, Artificial Sweeteners
- Omega-6 Vegetable Oils
- Dairy, depending on your ability to digest lactose and tolerate casein
- Nightshades
- Alcohol
- Antibiotics

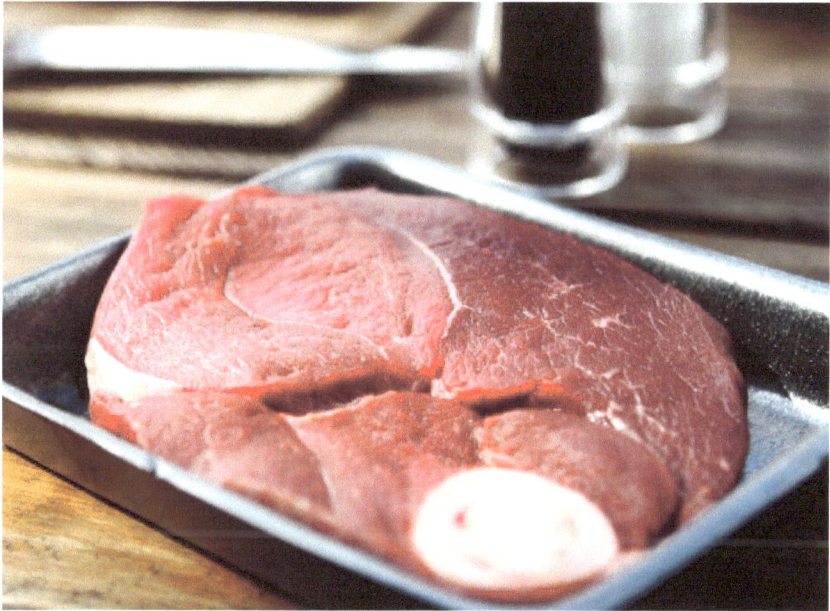

Image: freepik.com

── 21. MENTAL HEALTH ──

Improvement in mood and reduced anxiety was something I personally noticed. It is also one of the most common things I hear. When you combine a diet that's rich in nutrients, essential for the brain and nervous system's neurotransmitters, all while eliminating molecules that are inflammatory and triggering in the body, you create a recipe for great mental clarity and calmness.

Remember from our previous section that your gut is your "second brain." It too is grateful and responds favorably when it is not under a bombardment of inflammatory, triggering compounds. This diet works extremely well to help heal this area for many through giving it relief and opportunity to recover from all the triggers.

Brain Nutrients

Nutritionally we know omega-3 fatty acids as well as B12, both almost exclusively found in ONLY animal foods, play a critical role in proper neurological function. It is estimated that 20% of plant-based eaters are iron deficient and we know iron plays a key role in the creation of the critical feel good neurotransmitters, dopamine and serotonin. [42]

Hormone Balance

Balanced adequate hormones will fuel energy and vitality. Our hormones are made from cholesterol. Cholesterol is not the enemy! *This Carnivore Diet is rich in high quality fat and dietary cholesterol, completely absent from the plant kingdom.*

Many of modern western diseases are linked to prolonged, elevated insulin levels. A diet high in fat, with minimal carbohydrates will lower insulin and provide your body with the fuel it needs to produce proper hormones. These are very difficult to get in sufficient amounts unless you're consuming adequate animal foods.

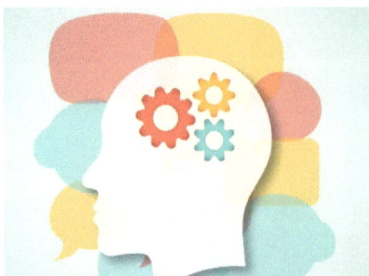

there were probably periods of time historically when humans did consume certain plant foods and carbohydrates, but those periods of indulgence were never year long, only seasonal.

22. VITAMIN C

One of the biggest concerns for those switching from a plant-based to an animal-based diet is that they will suffer a lack of vitamin C. It's one of the only nutrients more prevalent in plant foods vs. animal foods.

Vitamin C plays a key role in recycling glutathione / vitamin E and the formation of collagen triple helix - a key to the body's repairing and creating of connective tissues.

Despite claims, there's quite a bit of conflicting evidence it **prevents** colds or strengthens the immune system. [100] It does, however, help with enzymatic production of some neurotransmitters which may indirectly support optimal immune function.

The recommended daily allowance (RDA) is 60 mg. Higher doses may lead to kidney stones, diarrhea and nausea.

But there are no cases in predominantly meat based tribes showing signs of scurvy, a condition due to lack of dietary vitamin C. Historically consumption of fresh meat was known by sailors to treat scurvy. Pirates and others who got scurvy ate diets mostly of dried foods and dried meats which would've drastically reduced water-soluble vitamin C.

The USDA lists fresh meat as containing no vitamin C at all. Ironically, they never tested meat for vitamin C when making this claim. *The fact is, anywhere there's collagen there's vitamin C. We know from recent reports that there actually is vitamin C in muscle meat.*

Another huge factor to consider is that the RDA requirements were largely formulated on a carbohydrate diet. We know that when humans shift into a ketogenic state these variables often change. Hormone receptivity often increases when blood sugar is

lowered.

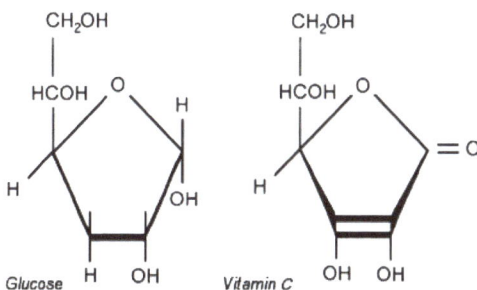

image.freepik.com

Vitamin C and Glucose are very similar biochemically. Glucose will compete with vitamin C on a carbohydrate driven metabolism, but when an individual is in a ketogenic state (high fat, low carb) glucose levels are lower, hence vitamin C needs become reduced.

We know from studies back in the early 20-30s that as little as 10mgs / day is more than enough to treat scurvy. Additionally these studies were largely done with individuals consuming a carbohydrate diet. Conclusion, we don't see Carnivores with scurvy today. We know that fresh meat will contain vitamin C and organs such as liver, even more. (100 grams / 4oz of beef liver contains 30% of the RDA of vitamin C).

━━━ 23. COFFEE & TEA ━━━

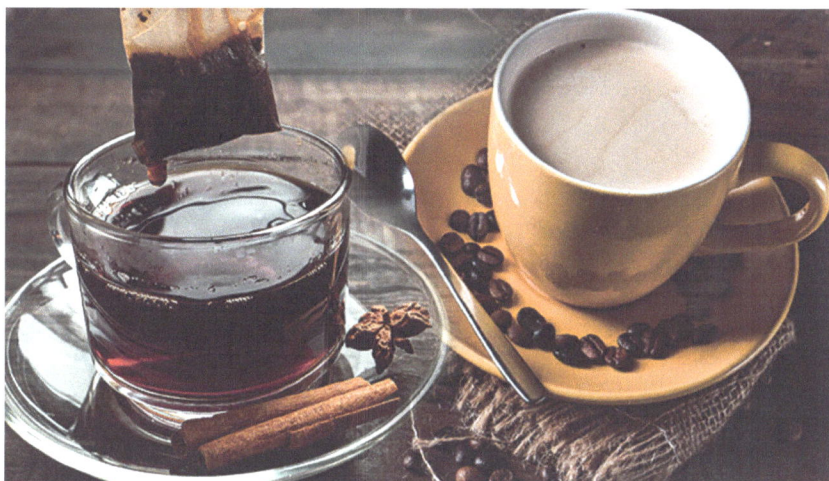
Image: Coffee and tea

Disclaimer - if you do well with coffee and really love your java, you can keep it. If we're strict Carnivore Diet, then both coffee and tea originate from plants and are technically not Carnivore. Both have compounds that may be harmful.

In animal models polyphenols, both high in coffee and tea have been shown to cause kidney damage, tumor growth and imbalance in their thyroid hormone levels. [63] [64]

In addition, both coffee and tea are mass produced and have a higher susceptibility to increased toxic molds and contaminants. I'm also a huge fan of optimized sleep. The caffeine in these beverages has an exceptional half life, meaning it can last well within your body for beyond 24 hours, impacting the quality of your sleep.

The Toxicity and Gut Issues

If you're new to Carnivore and you really like your coffee / tea, then don't attempt to tackle it all at once. But given the mold, potential toxicity, polyphenols, anxiety and environmental damage of monocropping and shipping these products, I do feel the trade off is a major benefit in almost all respects.

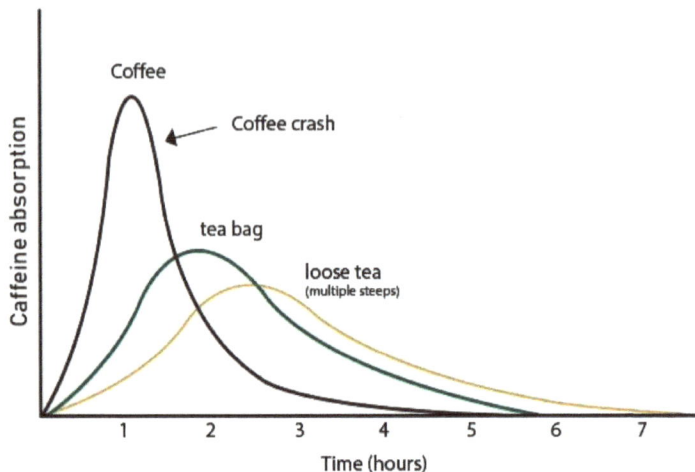

Image Source: Half-life difference caffeine sources [58]

Sleep

Depending on your caffeine metabolism, body size and how much you consume, you may be trying to wind down with a significant amount of caffeine still in your system. I've done personal experiments and talked with several others who have tracked significant reductions in REM sleep. This is the sleep that makes you feel mentally alert and rested. It aids in your ability to process the information and properly integrate learning and experiences.

I quit coffee a year ago. It was a painful addiction. I loved the taste, how I felt, everything about it mhh.. I loved the experience of sipping it in the mornings and adding in that delicious butter. After a few days of withdrawal headaches, lower energy, alertness and cravings, I was blown away at how much deeper I was sleeping. I was waking up so much more refreshed and my anxiety was significantly reduced. I was falling asleep quicker and much deeper.

If it's been a while since you've given yourself a caffeine break, maybe give it a try? See how you feel. You might find the trade off and increase in sleep quality outweighs the jolt and cycle of feeling buzzed, then drained. *I personally have noticed my energy is more steady and less anxious being caffeine free.*

Taking L-theanine in combination with stimulants like coffee and tea can help curb an overly anxious response to their effects. I find personally that it's a good addition for me whenever I'm trying out a new nootropic stack or supplement that may super-charge my energy.

24. WEIGHT LOSS

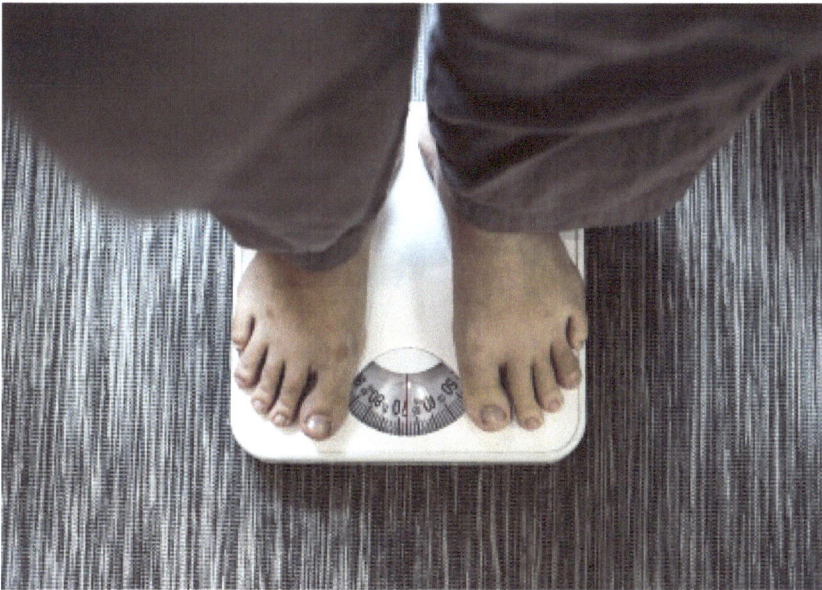

Image: freepik.com

The Carnivore Diet is exceptional at assisting in this goal. When writing this book, I wrote it from a place of treating anxiety, gut issues and optimizing my mental state. I personally have never dealt with real issues around weight loss. But I realize for many this is a very serious challenge and something that impacts their entire health so I decided to add a small section on the topic.

The biggest mistake I see people make is treating losing weight as simply restricting calories. They look at the calories in / calories out (CICO) model of weight loss and think, "well, if I just reduce portions I'm consuming I will be eating less calories while doing the same things and viola, I will lose weight." But that's a flawed way of looking at this.

Your body was intelligently designed to conserve and modulate your metabolism and energy expenditure based on your eating frequency, consumption and types of foods. For millions of years we experienced periods of inconsistent food supplies. It wasn't until the last 20-30,000 years that humans invented farming and then further invented food preservation methods to support chronic food consumption.

If you simply lower calorie intake your body is going to do what it's done for millions of years, lower your basal metabolic rate and slow down energy consumption, expenditure and reprioritize hormones signaling systems to slow down for survival. It's not going to go, "he's eating less, let's burn off all this fat and leave him with no energy reserves to survive." It's literally going to shift into a survival mode of not knowing when the next meal is and down regulate hormones.

Hormones

The body must tightly regulate blood sugar to prevent vessel, nerve and organ damage. When blood sugar climbs too high it can cause major internal damage. One of the primary ways it does this is to signal to your pancreas beta cells a need to release insulin.

Insulin

Insulin tells your body's fat storing cells to open up and accept the excess sugar so it can be normalized in the bloodstream. The cells open up and are stuffed with energy. When insulin is elevated the body stores excess food as fat and those fat cells (the stubborn extra fat you want to "melt" away) are receiving the exact opposite signal of utilizing their fat reserves to allow you to trim down.

To add insult to injury, when fat cells are stuffed, your body releases a hormone called Leptin. But when insulin levels are chronically elevated from refined carbs and processed food consumption, the cells are getting filled and releasing much more Leptin than normal. Hormone receptors for the "no longer hungry hormone" Leptin lose their sensitivity and those same foods no longer satiete and make you feel full. As a result you eat even more.

Hormone receptor sensitivity isn't just confined to insulin and leptin. Whenever hormones are impacted out of normal levels either elevated or reduced we see receptivity vary. For example, T3 Thyroid hormone is often reduced on ketogenic diets, yet we don't see reports of lowered energy from folks on those diet types. In fact, sports scientists have started to understand this and have engineered doping performance enhancing SARMs (Selective androgen receptor modulators) molecules that directly target the receptors for Testosterone as well as Human Growth Hormone for example to improve athletic performance, recovery and strength.

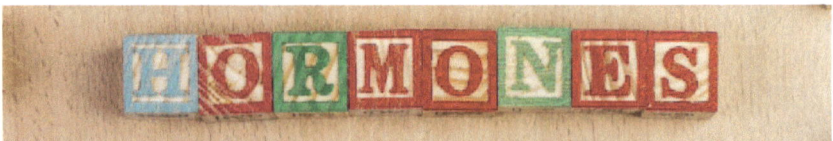

Image: freepik.com

What we must understand **to lose weight is that our hormones are the ultimate guide** to changing body composition. And this is largely impacted by the quality and macronutrient content of the food we're eating.

If you're on a Carnivore Diet you are shifting your body from a state of glucose fuel as a source, to a state of fat as your primary fuel. Because this diet is low carb, low glycemic and fuels us with all the essential nutrients and building blocks for healthy hormones, we see reduced insulin, increased energy and vitality and proper balance and receptivity of hormone signaling.

With the right balance of hormones you no longer feel hungry and continually eat. Your body is no longer receiving a signal to store fat, when you want to burn fat and overall energy levels can be normalized. It's a huge win all around when you can remove the foods that cause these issues.

If you want to learn more about this process I discuss more about this in my [Youtube channel](#) in some of my videos "weight loss" to help explain further.

Suffice it to say, weight loss can be quite significant and painless if your way of eating is aligned with nature and you're giving your body signals that you're in optimal health, eating foods it's evolved to consume. Combining a well constructed Carnivore Diet with daily movement, sunlight, intermittent fasting and high quality sleep will bring phenomenal results to the vast majority of people looking for relief in this area of their life.

25. LOWERING INFLAMMATION
AND AUTOIMMUNE

Inflammation itself isn't inherently all bad. It's a process we need our bodies to effectively do and manage. It only becomes an issue when we have chronic, elevated levels. Unfortunately our diets and lifestyle habits like smoking and alcohol consumption can all contribute to consistent elevated levels.

Combine that with plant molecules innately designed to fend off and kill predators, and you get a recipe for inflammation. Plants are high in omega-6 fatty acids which promote inflammation. They are loaded with many triggering compounds that trigger our immune response and invite inflammation.

All of this is going to contribute to elevated inflammation which when consistent, is a recipe for disaster in terms of how one is going to feel and their overall health.

Autoimmune

This is a condition in which the body's immune system attacks and damages its own tissues. Until we started understanding how critical nutrition is to our health and wellness and the cause of these issues, traditional medicine has stated that this happens for no reason.

The body is intelligently designed and I don't buy that it is attacking itself for no reason. There's definitely something happening for a reason. Traditional medicine treats the symptoms by suppressing the body's immune system. Just like we see with people taking antihistamines, rather than focus on the source and remove the histamine triggering foods, fuel the body with ways to lower histamine naturally through fueling our kidneys and diamine oxidase, we block the immune response and illicit a whole slew of side effects, along with weakening the immune function.

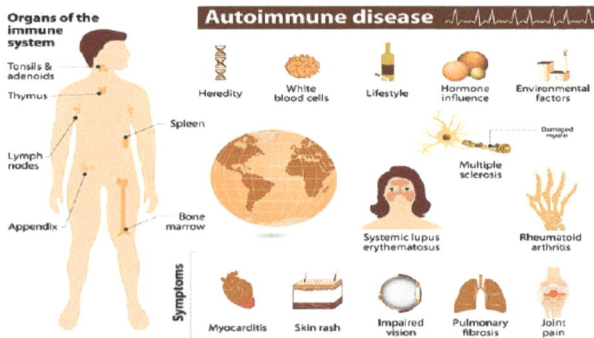

Autoimmune disease

Organs of the immune system: Tonsils & adenoids, Thymus, Spleen, Lymph nodes, Appendix, Bone marrow

Heredity, White blood cells, Lifestyle, Hormone influence, Environmental factors, Multiple sclerosis, Damaged myelin, Systemic lupus erythematosus, Rheumatoid arthritis

Symptoms: Myocarditis, Skin rash, Impaired vision, Pulmonary fibrosis, Joint pain

The following is a list of common, though perhaps not exhaustive, conditions caused by autoimmunity: Arthritis, Lupus, Celiac disease, Sjorgren's syndrome, polymyalgia, multiple sclerosis, Ankylosing spondylitis, Type 1 diabetes, Alopecia areata, Vasculitis and Temporal arteritis.

This is perhaps one of the most powerful things we see in the Carnivore community. Individuals with varying autoimmune disorders and diseases coming back from their proverbial graves, to thrive. Data is still new and we have studies and trials to conduct, but the anecdotes are powerful.

Elimination of the plant molecules that trigger inflammation will also cater to supporting a healthy biology lowering auto-immunity. As we mentioned in the graphics above, each of the respective plant molecules can trigger human bodies and have a serious impact on our immune systems and their response.

Along with the several conditions we've mentioned here in this text, we've seen drastic improvements from people with addiction, apnea, arthritis, asthma, depression, cardiovascular health, dental health, diabetes, digestion, joint pain, respiratory, sex, skin, sleep, fatigue, and weight loss. Literally 1000s of people dealing with these issues for years are coming out sharing their story of getting off symptom numbing medications and taking back their health.

26. ENHANCERS AND FAQS

There are certain sections and questions I want to address, but due to the scope of the book, and my wanting to keep it fairly tight in content, have held back.

Below is a list of a few things I find powerful in combination with the diet to ancestrally align and get to optimal health.

Carnivore Diet, ancestral enhancers:

1. Optimize Light

A. Get UVA/UVB from the sun, 30 mins / day for most people will be sufficient. As you tan, get more. If you live north, consider tanning. I talk in great detail about this in my light guide.

B. Eliminate blue/artificial light from your environment before sunrise and after sunset. This will drastically improve your sleep quality.

C. Consider photobiomodulation. Also known as red light therapy. This can help with skin collagen, hair regrowth, injuries and testosterone.

D. Infrared saunas for sweating and heating up from the inside out. Detoxing heavy metals, plastics, waste that accumulates in the body.

2. Optimize Sleep

A. Respect your rhythm and timing.

B. Eliminate stimulants from your diet, they hurt your sleep and REM.

C. Set up a cool, very dark, comfortable, safe, cozy sleeping situation.

D. Getting sunlight during the day will assist.

E. Restrict larger meals 3-4 hours prior to bedtime.

3. Get Steps In

A. Walking is very under-rated. Our ancestors and many extremely healthy preindustrial societies of today walk 5+ miles / day. Yet we rarely walk this much even in a week. Develop a habit of walking outside. I personally like to do so every morning to catch some morning sunshine in my eyes. I also enjoy it after a meal and it aids in digestion.

4. Consider Environmental Hermetics

A.   These are stressors from environmental elements, not plant molecules.

B.   Cold plunges, hot saunas, and exercising (this goes w/out saying).

C.   Cold exposure can make a major impact on sleep, mood and fat loss.

D.   Heat exposure is shown to reduce all cause mortality. It can assist with detoxification, cardiovascular health and stimulating more HGH.

5. Intermittent Fasting (IF), Fasting, Time-Restricted Feeding

A.   These are powerful tools, especially for metabolic resets and weight loss.

B.   If you're healthy and feeling up for it, consider tightening the time you eat throughout your day to a more limited, smaller window of hours.

C.   For example, you may want to skip breakfast and simply eat noon - 6pm, this would be intermittent fasting with a 6 hour window of eating.

D.   Restricting down your eating window will allow the body to reset and metabolically it can allow for many mechanisms of recovery to kick in.

Carnivore Diet FAQs

1.   If I'm a runner can I follow this way of eating?

-   Zach Bitter is an American Ultra Marathon runner who is Carnivore and currently holds the world record for the most distance 104.8 miles run in 12 hours. He's also the world record holder by more than 10 minutes of the world's fastest 100 mile run. For endurance and performance Carnivore is likely unmatched.

-   Sprinting may be a different case, but then again we don't have much information to support or sustain whether or not sprinting (or the amount of sprinting) is dependent and/or improved with carb consumption.

2. Does Carnivore work for CrossFit or Bodybuilding?

- This way of eating is ancestral. CrossFit competitions and Bodybuilding are likely things our ancestral bodies didn't experience with the same frequency we see today. I've talked with individuals who participate in these sports and carbs can often help them depending on their goals and demands. Though it's possible I think if you're interested and focused on this level of fitness, I would consider incorporating targeted carbs of high quality such as tubers like sweet potatoes at certain times pre/post exercise.

- For most standard weight lifting activities I do just fine working 2-3 muscle groups for 45-60 minutes.

3. Are my favorite foods gone forever? Will I ever be able to enjoy coffee, chocolate, a delicious salad?

- The power of this diet is the elimination aspect. After you've done Carnivore and you've started to see and feel just how healthy you can get, I think you'll be much less concerned with indulging in foods that may negatively impact you. Cravings also subside drastically after passing that first 4-5 weeks of no longer consuming that food type.

- I do realize others such as family and friends may tempt you to partake of those food types. And you are more than welcome to try them. Just try smaller than usual portions, and try your best to titrate (limit and then pause) consumption to see how your body reacts.

- If you can consume chocolate and then wait 2-3 days and do not notice any ill effects I would reintroduce once again and then wait another 2-3 days before confirming if it's truly tolerable and okay for you.

- People have reached out concerned they may never be able to eat their cheesecake or tomato pasta. For most I believe you'll become more sensitive but not less tolerating of triggering foods. Your baseline inflammation and vitality will be more clear. If it makes you sick, you'll feel it more and if you have big enough goals and desires, consuming harmful foods shouldn't be a concern.

▬ 27. CONCLUSION ▬

In writing this text I never intended it to grow to this size. My coach and colleagues told me it was enough at 75 pages, but I kept wanting to add more things.

I kept listening, searching and seeking for answers to all the concerns and counterpoints I felt most skeptical about. I wanted to leave no stone unturned and really build a convincing argument to instill unwavering confidence in those who want to take this journey.

I'm grateful for this process and all the help I received from the coach and teams. I believe the work of this text, along with brilliant minds of several close friends and colleagues, is transforming the way we are looking at and treating human disease, as well as enhancing ourselves to the most optimal versions.

Conditions such as anxiety or depression do not have to be a life sentence. Being overweight does not have to be what happens as you get older.

Our environment, both outside of our bodies as well INSIDE ourselves (the things we allow to enter our mouths and go into our gut and intestines to be absorbed), play a critical role in how we think, feel, act and experience our lives.

Human beings can absolutely thrive through consuming higher quantities of higher quality, more bioavailable, less toxic animal foods. Removing foods that hurt us, that are unnatural and providing the nutrition our ancestors were biologically evolved to thrive with, will make us better, more effective, more optimal, healthier and more connected. Connected to nature, to our own bodies and to the delicate and beautiful life cycle of this planet.

Online you will find much more of my content at karnivorekurt.com. You can follow me on Instagram @karnivorekurt and subscribe to our Youtube channel to watch videos of what I'm learning and teaching each week.

Lastly, I just want to THANK YOU. I want to thank you for taking the initiative to care enough to invest in yourself and your vitality. I realize it's an incredible challenge for most of us and it takes tremendous effort.

Many of you may not be coming from as dark a place, or perhaps the place you're coming from is much darker than mine was. Either way, I realize it can take an inhuman amount of courage, tremendous effort and perseverance to overcome habit gravity, to climb out of that hole and disrupt the old habits and thinking that has landed so many in our society in places of health crisis.

I look forward to hearing and seeing all the success stories to come. Thank you.

─ **28. REFERENCES** ─

01   Watson, K. (2019, October 16). Type 3 Diabetes and Alzheimer's Disease: What You Need to Know. https://www.healthline.com/health/type-3-diabetes

02   Eldredge, S. and Biek, B. (2019, September). Glad you asked: Ice Ages - What are they and what causes them? https://geology.utah.gov/map-pub/survey-notes/glad-you-asked/ice-ages-what-are-they-and-what-causes-them/

03   Miki, B.D., Avi, G., Israel, H. & Ran, B. (2011, December 9). Man the Fat Hunter: The Demise of Homo erectus and the Emergence of a New Hominin Lineage in the Middle Pleistocene (ca. 400 kyr) Levant. https://journals.plos.org/plosone/article?id=10.1371/journal.pone.0028689

04   Pobiner, B. (2016, February 23). Human Nature The First Butchers Were there other toolmakers and meat eaters in our family tree? https://www.sapiens.org/evolution/homo-sapiens-and-tool-making/

05   United States Food & Drug Administration. (2018, January 04). Consumer Info About Food from Genetically Engineered Plants. https://www.fda.gov/food/food-new-plant-varieties/consumer-info-about-food-genetically-engineered-plants

06   John, T. (2016, June 27). Many native cultures have high-carb diets and are healthy. It's the quality of the carbs they eat! https://johntropea.tumblr.com/post/146554890386/many-native-cultures-have-high-carb-diets-and-are

07   Harriman, C. (2017, August 1). Pulling ancel keys out from under the bus. https://oldwayspt.org/blog/pulling-ancel-keys-out-under-bus

08   Team Asprey. (2018, April 27). 4 Top Antinutrients To Avoid - And Why. https://blog.daveasprey.com/4-top-antinutrients-to-avoid-and-why/

09   The National Kidney Foundation. (n.d.). Calcium Oxalate Stones. https://www.kidney.org/atoz/content/calcium-oxalate-stone

10   National Center for Complementary and Integrative Health. (2019, October 09). 7 Things To Know About Omega-3 Fatty Acids. https://nccih.nih.gov/health/tips/omega

11   Simopoulos, A.P. (2002, October). The importance of the ratio of omega-6/omega-3 essential fatty acids. https://www.ncbi.nlm.nih.gov/pubmed/1244290

12   Simopoulos, A.P. (2016, March). An Increase in the Omega-6/Omega-3 Fatty Acid Ratio Increases the Risk for Obesity. https://www.ncbi.nlm. nih.gov/pmc/articles/PMC4808858/

13   Gester, H. (1998). Can adults adequately convert alpha-linolenic acid (18:3n-3) to eicosapentaenoic acid (20:5n-3) and docosahexaenoic acid (22:6n-3). https://www.ncbi.nlm.nih.gov/pubmed/9637947

14   Tang, G. (2010, May). Bioconversion of dietary provitamin A carotenoids to vitamin A in humans1,2,3,4,5. https://www.ncbi.nlm.nih.gov/pmc/ articles/PMC2854912/

15   Sisson, Mark. (n.d.). Is Iron the New Cholesterol? https://www.marksdailyapple.com/is-iron-the-new-cholesterol/

16   Vitamin D. (2018, November). https://www.hormone.org/your-health-and-hormones/glands-and-hormones-a-to-z/hormones/vitamin-d

17   Lindqvist, P. G., Epstein, E., Nielsen, K., Landin☐Olsson, M., Ingvar, C. & Olsson, H. (2016, March 16). Avoidance of sun exposure as a risk factor for major causes of death: a competing risk analysis of the Melanoma in Southern Sweden cohort. https://onlinelibrary.wiley. com/doi/full/10.1111/joim.12496

18   Veerman, J.L., Healy, G.N., Cobiac, L.J., Vos, T., Wrinkler, E., Owen, N. & Dunstan, D.W.(2012, December 01). Television viewing time and reduced life expectancy: a life table analysis. https://bjsm.bmj.com/ content/46/13/927

19   Ferrières, J. (2004, January). The French paradox: lessons for other countries. https://www.ncbi.nlm.nih.gov/pmc/articles/PMC1768013/

20   Wang, Z., Klipfell, E., Bennett, B. et al. Gut flora metabolism of phosphatidylcholine promotes cardiovascular disease. Nature 472, 57–63 (2011). https://www.nature.com/articles/nature09922

21   Gran P. & Cameron-Smith D. (2011, June 25). The actions of exogenous leucine on mTOR signalling and amino acid transporters in human myotubes. https://www.ncbi.nlm.nih.gov/pmc/articles/ PMC3141572/

22   Aykan N.F. (2015, December 28). Red Meat and Colorectal Cancer. https://www.ncbi.nlm.nih.gov/pmc/articles/PMC4698595/

23   Perfect Keto Staff. (2018, August 22). The 7 Benefits of Grass Fed Beef: The Nutritional Powerhouse. https://perfectketo.com/benefits-of-grass-fed-beef/

24   Stephen, T. (2020, January). Stephen improved his muscle mass, digestion, and skin on a carnivore diet. https://meatrx.com/category/success-stories/

25   Sources of Greenhouse Gas Emissions. (n.d.). https://www.epa.gov/ghgemissions/sources-greenhouse-gas-emissions

26   Eckelman, M.J. & Sherman, J. (2016, June 9). Environmental Impacts of the U.S. Health Care System and Effects on Public Health. https://journals.plos.org/plosone/article?id=10.1371/journal.pone.0157014

27   Peter Ballerstedt blog. https://twitter.com/GrassBased

28   Management Must Be Holistic. (n.d.). https://www.savory.global/holistic-management/

29   White Oak Pastures Team. (2019, June). Study: White Oak Pastures Beef Reduces Atmospheric Carbon. http://blog.whiteoakpastures.com/blog/carbon-negative-grassfed-beef

30   Boerama, A., Peeters, A., Swolfs, S., Vandevenne, F., Jacobs, S., Staes, J. & Miere, P. (2016, May 31). Soybean Trade: Balancing Environmental and Socio-Economic Impacts of an Intercontinental Market. https://www.ncbi.nlm.nih.gov/pmc/articles/PMC4887031/

31   Triune brain. (2020, January 27). https://en.wikipedia.org/wiki/Triune_brain

32   Beware of This Home Cooking Pitfall. (n.d.) https://cookware.mercola.com/ceramic-cookware.aspx

33   Endocrine Disruptors. (2020, January 20). https://www.niehs.nih.gov/health/topics/agents/endocrine/index.cfm

34   Young, L.B, (2018, March 28). The Science Behind a Soda Can. https://www.reagent.co.uk/the-science-behind-a-soda-can/

35 Martin, W.F., Armstrong, L.E. and Rodriguez, N.R. (2005, September 20). Dietary protein intake and renal function. https://www.ncbi.nlm.nih.gov/pmc/articles/PMC1262767/

36 Meat Heals. (2019, November 01). Michael improved his mood/mental health, skin, vision, and weight loss, and treated his addiction, arthritis, chronic fatigue, and GERD on a carnivore diet. https://meatrx.com/category/success-stories/arthritis/

37 Allergy Facts. (2018, September 01). https://acaai.org/news/facts-statistics/allergies

38 The Food List. (n.d.). https://www.histamineintolerance.org.uk/about/the-food-diary/the-food-list/

39 Ho, K.S., Tan, C.Y., Mohd Daud, M.A. & Seow-Choen, F. (2012, September 07). Stopping or reducing dietary fiber intake reduces constipation and its associated symptoms. https://www.ncbi.nlm.nih.gov/pmc/articles/PMC3435786/

40 Peery, A.F., Barrett, P.R., Park, D., Rogers, A.J., Galanko, J.A., Martin, C.F. & Sandler R.S. (2012, February). A high-fiber diet does not protect against asymptomatic diverticulosis. https://www.ncbi.nlm.nih.gov/pubmed/22062360

41 Farvid, M.S., Eliassen, H.A, Cho, E., Liao, X., Chen, W.Y. & Willett, W.C. (2016, February). Dietary Fiber Intake in Young Adults and Breast Cancer Risk. https://pediatrics.aappublications.org/content/early/2016/01/28/peds.2015-1226

42 Kim, J., Wessling-Resnick, M. (2014, August 02). Iron and Mechanisms of Emotional Behavior. https://www.ncbi.nlm.nih.gov/pmc/articles/PMC4253901/

43 Poortmans, J.R. & Dellalieux, O. (2000, March). Do regular high protein diets have potential health risks on kidney function in athletes? https://www.ncbi.nlm.nih.gov/pubmed/10722779

44   Walser, M. (1999). 7 Effects of Protein Intake on Renal Function and on the Development of Renal Disease. https://www.ncbi.nlm.nih.gov/books/NBK224634/

45   Chris Palmer MD. (2020). Retrieved from https://www.chrispalmermd.com/

46   Connor, S. (2013, June 26). Throwing ability 'helped turn humans from second-rate primate into most successful species on the planet'. https://www.independent.co.uk/news/science/throwing-ability-helped-turn-humans-from-second-rate-primate-into-most-successful-species-on-the-8675395.html

47   E.Y, (2019, May 18). Meat Consumption Growth in Hong Kong is Alarming. https://medium.com/@ecyY/meat-consumption-growth-in-hong-kong-is-alarming-872e46bf40ca?

28   Sussman, D., van Eede, M., Wong, M.D., Adamson, S.L. & Henkelman, M. (2013, May 08). Effects of a ketogenic diet during pregnancy on embryonic growth in the mouse. https://www.ncbi.nlm.nih.gov/pubmed/23656724

49   Emotional eating. (2020, January 13). https://en.wikipedia.org/wiki/Emotional_eating

50   Curhan, G.C. (2019, May 28). Interpretation of kidney stone composition analysis.https://www.uptodate.com/contents/interpretation-of-kidney-stone-composition-analysis

51   Newman, T. (2018, September 05). Anxiety in the West: Is it on the rise? https://www.medicalnewstoday.com/articles/322877.php#1

52   Gray, N. (2016, December 09). The double edged sword: High does of polyphenols may damage DNA. https://www.nutraingredients.com/Article/2016/12/09/The-double-edged-sword-High-doses-of-polyphenols-may-damage-DNA#

53   Shmerling, R.H. (2017, September 25). The latest scoop on the health benefits of coffee. https://www.health.harvard.edu/blog/the-latest-scoop-on-the-health-benefits-of-coffee-2017092512429

54   Saxena, A. (2019, January 24). Women who eat meat less prone to disease: study.
https://indianexpress.com/article/lifestyle/health/women-who-eat-meat-less-prone-to-disease-study-5553067/

55   Kay, G.G. (2000, June). The effects of antihistamines on cognition and performance.
https://www.jacionline.org/article/S0091-6749(00)79554-6/fulltext

56   corpdetoxbliss. (2018, January 08). Optimum Health! Are we treating the symptoms or the Cause? [Blog post]. Retrieved from https://steemit.com/health/@corpdetoxbliss/optimum-health-are-we-treating-the-symptoms-or-the-cause

57   Folic acid. (2019, April 01). https://www.womenshealth.gov/a-z-topics/folic-acid

58   Tea Caffeine Guide. (2015, April 06).
https://www.teasenz.com/chinese-tea/tea-caffeine.html

59   Beef, grass-fed, strip steaks, lean only, raw Nutrition Facts & Calories. (n.d.).
https://nutritiondata.self.com/facts/beef-products/10525/2

60   Jensen, R.G. (1999, December). Lipids in human milk.
https://www.ncbi.nlm.nih.gov/pubmed/10652985

61   Navarrete, A., van Schaik, C.P., Isler, K. (2011, November). Energetics and the evolution of human brain size. https://www.ncbi.nlm.nih.gov/pubmed/22080949

62   Ho, K.S., Tan, C.Y., Mohd Daud, M.A. & Seow-Choen, F. (2012, September 07). Stopping or reducing dietary fiber intake reduces constipation and its associated symptoms. https://www.ncbi.nlm.nih.gov/pmc/articles/PMC3435786/

63   Cory, H., Passarelli, S., Szeto, J., Tamez, M. & Mattei1, J. (2018, September 21). The Role of Polyphenols in Human Health and Food Systems: A Mini-Review. https://www.ncbi.nlm.nih.gov/pmc/articles/PMC6160559/

64   Mennen, L.I., Walker, R., Bennetau-Pelissero, C. & Scalbert, A. (2005, January). Risks and safety of polyphenol consumption. https://www.ncbi. nlm.nih.gov/pubmed/15640498

65   Compound Interest. (2017, June 07). The Chemistry of Allergies and Antihistamines. http://scitechconnect.elsevier.com/the-chemistry-of-allergies-and-antihistamines/

66   Huizen, J. (2018, July 23). Which foods are high in histamine? https://www.medicalnewstoday.com/articles/322543.php

67   Carnivore Aurelius.(2019). The 10 Biggest Vegan Diet Lies (Debunked). [Blog post]. Retrieved from https://carnivoreaurelius.com/vegan-diet-debunked/

68   Stock, K. (2018, May 29). Do you need fiber? https://www.kevinstock.io/health/do-you-need-fiber/

69   Is Fiber Bad For You? The Top 12 Myths And The Real Truth About Whether Fiber Is Killing Your Insides. (n.d.). https://bengreenfieldfitness.com/article/nutrition-articles/is-fiber-bad-for-you/

70   Norman, A. (2008, August 01). From vitamin D to hormone D: fundamentals of the vitamin D endocrine system essential for good health. https://academic.oup.com/ajcn/article/88/2/491S/4649916

71   Is there a difference between L-methylfolate and folic acid supplementation for patients with the MTHFR C677T mutation? (n.d.) https://genesight.com/is-there-a-difference-between-l-methylfolate-and-folic-acid-supplementation-for-patients-with-the-mthfr-c677t-mutation/

72   Perfect Keto Staff. (2018, October 26). Ketosis During Pregnancy. https://perfectketo.com/ketosis-during-pregnancy/

73   Rosenbloom, C. (2019, April 09). The dangers of a keto diet in pregnancy. https://www.todaysparent.com/pregnancy/keto-pregnancy-is-not-a-healthy-choice

74   Emmerich, M. (2012, January 26). Keto During Pregnancy. https://mariamindbodyhealth.com/keto-pregnancy/

75 Mullens, A. (2019, October 25). Is low carb and keto safe during pregnancy? https://www.dietdoctor.com/low-carb/pregnancy

76 KenDBerryMD. (2018, December 10). Is the Ketogenic Diet Safe in Pregnancy? (Very Important). [Video File]. Retrived from https://www.youtube.com/watch?v=Kv2RVFxtgFA

77 Colino, S. (2019, January 08). Can the Keto Diet Help Boost Fertility? https://www.ccrmivf.com/news-events/keto-diet/

78 Ciccarelli, L. (2018, August 25). Keto and PCOS: How a Ketogenic Diet Helps Polycystic Ovarian Syndrome. https://perfectketo.com/keto-pcos/

79 Rachel. (2018, August 20). Here's What Research Says About Keto While Breastfeeding. https://perfectketo.com/keto-while-breastfeeding/

80 English, A. (2016, June 07). Part One: Understanding Heuristics and Biases in Homeland Security: The Triune Brain. https://medium.com/homeland-security/part-one-understanding-heuristics-and-biases-in-homeland-security-the-triune-brain-d374317f508

81 Phineas Gage. (2020, January 28). https://en.wikipedia.org/wiki/Phineas_Gage

82 Orenstein, B. (2017, September 27). Is Your Diet Giving You Diarrhea? https://www.everydayhealth.com/diarrhea-management-photos/diarrhea-and-diet.aspx

83 Rafi, Z. (2019, Jun 27). How TMAO Fooled Us. Retrieved from https://lesslikely.com/nutrition/tmao-mendelian-randomization/

84 mTOR. (2020, January 03). https://en.m.wikipedia.org/wiki/MTOR

85 Kresser, C. (2019, June 17). Myths and Truths About Fiber. https://chriskresser.com/myths-and-truths-about-fiber/

86 stroids. (2007, December 05). How long does the average cow spend eating each day? [Online discussion group]. Retrieved from https://www.funtrivia.com/askft/Question89449.html

87   Carnivore Aurelius.(2019). Grass-Fed vs. Grain-Fed: 10 Things You Need To Consider. [Blog post]. Retrieved from https://carnivoreaurelius.com/grass-fed-vs-grain-fed/

88   Saladino, P. (m.d.). Is Grass-Fed Meat Really Worth It? https://carnivoremd.com/is-grass-fed-meat-really-worth-it/

89   Carnivore Aurelius.(2019). Carnivore Diet: Everything You Need To Know (Updated 2020). https://carnivoreaurelius.com/carnivore-diet/

90   Carnivore Aurelius.(2019). The Science of Saponins: 5 Dangers of Eating Them. https://carnivoreaurelius.com/saponins/

91   O'Hearn, A.L. (2017, February 21). C is for Carnivore. http://www.empiri.ca/2017/02/c-is-for-carnivore.html

92   Kim, J. & Wessling-Resnick, M. (2014, August 2). Iron and Mechanisms of Emotional Behavior. https://www.ncbi.nlm.nih.gov/pmc/articles/PMC4253901/

93   Monsen, E.R. (1988, July). Iron nutrition and absorption: dietary factors which impact iron bioavailability. https://www.ncbi.nlm.nih.gov/pubmed/3290310

94   Spritzler, F. (2017, May 15). 12 Natural Ways to Balance Your Hormones. https://www.healthline.com/nutrition/balance-hormones#section1

95   Watson, S. (2019, March 21). Autoimmune Diseases: Types, Symptoms, Causes, and More. https://www.healthline.com/health/autoimmune-disorders

96   Underwood, E. (2018, September 20). Your gut is directly connected to your brain, by a newly discovered neuron circuit. https://www.sciencemag.org/news/2018/09/your-gut-directly-connected-your-brain-newly-discovered-neuron-circuit

97   Campos, M. (2018, October 18). What is keto flu? https://www.health.harvard.edu/blog/what-is-keto-flu-2018101815052

98   Ballerstedt, P. (2019, October). No, eating animal source foods won't ruin the planet! [PDF File]. Retrieved from https://drive.google.com/file/d/1aOjLad9BsOUDDXvf3h1Jz9O_tzkux_8h/view

99   NFE2L2. (2019, November 10). https://en.wikipedia.org/wiki/NFE2L2

DISCLAIMER

The author and contributors of Kurt Yazici's The Carnivore Diet and anyone associated with Crushvertise. are not doctors or other medical health professionals. The information, including but not limited to, text, graphics, images and other material contained in this e-book publication and which may be found on the website karnivorekurt.com are for general education and informational purposes only. This publication and the website karnivorekurt.com are not intended to be a substitute for professional medical advice, diagnosis or treatment. Always seek the advice of your physician or other qualified healthcare provider with any questions you may have regarding your pregnancy or any other medical condition or treatment you may have and before undertaking a new health care regimen, diet (including, supplements and herbal or nutritional treatments), or exercise program. Never disregard professional medical advice or delay in seeking it because of something you have read in this publication or on karnivorekurt.com. Reliance on any information appearing in this publication or on karnivorekurt.com is solely at your own risk. Developments in medical research may impact the information that may appear in this publication and on karnivorekurt.com. The author assumes no duty to update the content to include the most recent information relevant to the content. If you are having a health emergency, call your health care professional, or 911 (in the United States), immediately. Copyright 2020. All rights reserved. No part of this book may be reproduced in any form without written permission from the author. Except by a reviewer who may quote brief passages in a review. Cover and Book Design by "Ritesh Suri and Cedric Mendoza".